POSITIVE AGING

POSITIVE AGING

A Guide for Mental
Health Professionals
and Consumers

ROBERT D. HILL

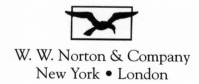

W. W. Norton & Company
New York • London

Figures by Kent Hepworth, graphic artist.

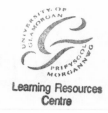

Copyright © 2005 by Robert D. Hill

For information about permission to reproduce selections from this book, write to Permissions, W. W. Norton & Company, Inc., 500 Fifth Avenue, New York, NY 10110

Production Manager: Leeann Graham
Composition by Pine Tree Composition, Inc.
Manufacturing by Quebecor World Fairfield Graphics

Library of Congress Cataloging-in-Publication Data

Hill, Robert D.
Positive aging : a guide for mental health professionals and consumers /
  Robert D. Hill.
    p. cm.
Includes bibliographical references and index.
ISBN 0-393-70453-X
1. Gerontology. 2. Older people—Health and hygiene. 3. Quality of life.
I. Title.

HQ1061.H53 2005
305.26—dc22   2004066278

W. W. Norton & Company, Inc., 500 Fifth Avenue, New York, N.Y. 10110
www.wwnorton.com

W. W. Norton & Company Ltd., Castle House, 75/76 Wells St., London
W1T 3QT

1 2 3 4 5 6 7 8 9 0

I express deep appreciation to my wife and longtime companion, Debra K. Hill, for her assistance in the preparation and editing of this book. This book is dedicated to my great aunt, C. Belle Grischow, who is 94 years old and a model of positive aging.

CONTENTS

INTRODUCTION

Characterizing the process of growing old represents a major social challenge in our modern era. Twentieth-century notions of human aging have previously been tied to retirement, senility, disability, and death. The elderly needed assistance in everyday living as they became less able to deal with the unavoidable consequences of old age. Older adults in the 20th century were separated from the mainstream of society as reluctant observers of social change. The stereotype of the older person who is preoccupied with his or her fears about old age has been pervasive. Macolm Cowley, who lived and died in the 20th century, described his own experience with aging in terms that are thematic of deterioration and obsolescence (Cowley, 1980).

> We don't have to read books in order to learn that one's eighties are a time of gradually narrowing horizons. . . . Trees on a not-so-distant hillside are no longer oaks or maples, but merely a blur. . . . Your steps are less assured, your sense of balance is faulty; soon you hesitate to venture beyond your own street. . . . Many of your old friends have vanished and it is harder to find new ones. . . . More and more the older person is driven back into himself; more and more he is occupied with what goes on in his mind. (pp. 54–55)

Age-related decline always has and always will be a part of growing old. Deteriorative processes yield predictable consequences including limitations, narrowing of horizons, disability, pain, and suffering.

The 21st century, however, is poised to teach us that old age can be much more than physical or cognitive decline. This new viewpoint has been catalyzed by the sociocultural trend of persons in first world countries who are living longer, and continuing to make contributions to society in their later years. The longevity of persons in the first world has been steadily increasing (by as much as two to five years per decade) and this trend will likely continue into the future. Today, for example, the average life span of men and women in the United States exceeds 76 years. This means that the average American can expect to live an active and purposeful life not only past the stereotypical 65-year age marker for retirement, but well into his or her seventh and eighth decade. An extended life span means that people are able to make more contributions to society in their later years. Many of the political, social, and religious leaders in our modern age have come from the ranks of the elderly, and these high-profile persons are optimistic role models of what aging is becoming in the 21st century.

Who we think of as "very old" is changing as well. One of the fastest growing groups in the United States are those living up to and beyond a hundred years. The number of centenarians has swelled to nearly 70,000 persons in the United States (Koplan & Fleming, 2000; Krach & Velkoff, 1999). And these have been eclipsed by a newly discovered small group of extremely long lived persons, supercentenarians, whose life span exceeds 109 years (Coles, 2004a, 2004b). It is difficult to know whether this longevity trend will continue into the future and how it will shape the average person's views of the aging process. However, what can be expected to change are the perceptions of quality of life that is possible, in our modern era, for people in their later years.

Even among those who are suffering from age-related chronic disability and disease, living into old and even very old age is a reality. Advances in the medical sciences and in geriatric care have not only extended life, but have created ways to help the older patient remain functional, even with a chronic disease. Whether in health or in disease, people expect to live beyond the age of retirement and to work, play, and make contributions to their family and community. Given these societal trends, new terms have emerged to capture the aging process.

Successful and *optimal* aging are labels that have made their way from the scientific literature to the general public to describe persons who are living into very old age and who experience a high quality of life in the process. The popularity of terms such as *successful aging* is shaping how people expect to grow old. Rowe and Kahn (1998) construed successful aging as an optimistic variant of the stereotypical aging experience. However, because successful aging connotes an ideal that few people will be able achieve (in fact, some scholars have estimated that less than 10% of the population could call themselves successful agers), new terms must emerge that capture the essence of old age with its obvious infirmities while still preserving the advantages of a positive outlook on later life.

The stage is set for elucidating new terms or ideas that capture a more optimistic view of human aging. The question arises, however, as to where such terminology will come from or what professional or scientific discipline is in the best position to champion innovative conceptualizations of growing old in the 21st century and the role of individual choice in taking full advantage of our increased longevity. It is also hoped that such an approach to labeling the aging experience could open the door to new understandings and directions for future research in gerontology and geropsychology.

The goal of this book is to promulgate a term that fits the 21st-century mindset about old age. "Positive Aging," as the title of this book implies, represents such an umbrella idea or a guiding framework for describing the challenges and opportunities that can be found in later life, and the role of individual choice in directing how one approaches growing old in this modern, life-extension era. This book will define the term *positive aging,* and describe why it is a valid conceptualization of a psychological approach to growing old that is distinct from other actuarially based terms such as *successful, normal,* and *diseased aging.*

The backdrop for positive aging comes from the positive psychology movement that has been recently popularized in the field of psychology. In an essay, Martin Seligman, a central figure in the positive psychology movement, noted:

The field of positive psychology at the subjective level is about valued subjective experiences: well-being, contentment, and satisfaction (in the past); hope and optimism (for the future); and flow and happiness (in the present). At the individual level, it is about positive individual traits: the capacity for love and vocation, courage, interpersonal skill, aesthetic sensibility, perseverance, forgiveness, originality, future mindedness, spirituality, high talent, and wisdom." (Seligman & Csikszentmihalyi, 2000, p. 1)

In Seligman's view the essence of positive psychology is, "a science that takes as its primary task the understanding of what makes life worth living" (Seligman & Csikszentmihalyi, 2000, p. 13). Among the many features of positive psychology that could have meaning for constructing a term descriptive of human aging in all of its forms and variations, is the focus on what a person is capable of doing, accomplishing, or overcoming, rather than on the passive avoidance of problems of living and the fear of pain, disability, and a restricted lifestyle in later life. Positive psychology, then, opens the door to new approaches to old problems and stereotypes of growing old. Without question aging is a period when physical decline is a visible and prominent aspect of living and a time during which one must cope with issues of cognitive decline in order to preserve quality of life. How one conceptualizes growing old in the presence or absence of disease, while still experiencing happiness and a positive sense of well-being, is descriptive of *positive aging*.

Terms that are consistent with positive aging have already begun to appear in the scientific literature. "Positive Spirituality," coined by Crowther and colleagues (Crowther, Parker, Achenbaum, Larimore, & Koenig, 2002) is an example of this phenomenon. Chapter 7 will describe positive spirituality and its relation to the overarching notion of positive aging as well as specific techniques that emerge from this framework that offer new ways to approach the problems and issues of growing old. Positive aging, in some respects, is more comprehensive than successful aging. In positive aging it is possible to experience, even in the presence of disease and infirmity, quality of life and a sense of well-being. As will be described in this book, a person who lives into (and beyond) the eighth decade of life is likely to experience decline in memory function as well as physical disability, disease, and a diminishment of his or her social network. It would seem, for example, that a home-bound 87-year-old adult who is suffering from chronic osteoporosis and has some memory impairment would *not* be a candidate for successful aging. However, such a person could consider him- or herself a positive ager because positive aging takes into account the possibility of finding quality of life, meaning, and completeness even when home-bound and ill. In essence, positive aging requires that a person make choices and engage in coping, even when experiencing the predictable physical and psychological limitations that are part of being old. Finding happiness and well-being in the aging process is similar to the meaning in Csikszentmihalyi's statement:

> Happiness is not something that happens. It is not the result of good fortune or random change. Happiness, in fact, is a condition that must be prepared for, cultivated, and defended privately by each person. People who learn to control inner experience will be able to determine the quality of their lives, which is as close as any of us can come to being happy. (Csikszentmihalyi, 1990, p. 2)

In this sense, positive aging, like happiness, is as much a state of mind as it is any specific form of action or strategy. To be happy and healthy in old age involves discipline in reframing perceptions and cultivating positive emotions to cope with the realistic dilemmas of aging.

The nine chapters of this book present different aspects of positive aging and tools that practitioners as well as geriatric counselors can use to help older adults maintain a positive aging outlook even in the presence of age-related decline. A brief description of each chapter follows:

Chapter 1, "A Framework for Positive Aging," provides a general overview and background for the term *positive aging*. Included is a description of the ways in which it is distinct from other terms that describe the aging process. A rationale is presented for utilizing positive aging to capture the psychological nature of growing old and the possibility to adopt lifestyle patterns and ways of thinking that can promote well-being in old age.

Chapter 2, "Three Life Span Models of Aging," describes models of adult development and aging that are supportive of positive aging: Erikson's Life Stages of Development; Continuity Theory; and

Selectivity, Optimization, and Compensation (SOC). A brief review of each theory is provided along with examples of how positive aging emerges from them.

Chapter 3, "Age-Related Decline and Its Effects," describes decline in old age and how terms such as *successful, normal, impaired,* and *diseased* aging are captured in trajectories of decline. The heterogeneity of normal aging is highlighted. Wisdom is described as a consequence of age-related change and as a life skill that can be acquired for achieving positive aging.

Chapter 4, "Assessment Strategies and Instruments," reviews assessment approaches for common old-age issues including cognitive deficits, depressive and anxious symptomatology, functional independence, and well-being and life satisfaction. The relationship between assessment and positive aging is examined.

Chapter 5, "Psychological Barriers to Positive Aging," describes maladaptive life span stylistics, including rigidity, negativity, worry, regret, and self-absorption, and how these represent barriers to positive aging. Techniques are presented for changing maladaptive stylistics in order to foster positive aging.

Chapter 6, "Psychotherapies and Special Populations," reviews several traditional psychotherapy modalities, including psychodynamic, behavioral and cognitive behavioral therapy, family systems, existential therapy, and group counseling, to address mental health concerns in old age. A positive aging strategy for addressing the needs of older adults from special populations is reviewed including those who represent diversity with respect to gender, race, sexual orientation, and socioeconomic status.

Chapter 7, "Positive Spirituality and Meaning-Based Counseling," examines the term *positive spirituality* and its relationship to positive aging. Strategies and techniques for mental health treatment of age-related issues and concerns that emerge from a positive spirituality/positive aging approach to living are examined. These meaning-based life span strategies include gratitude, forgiveness, and altruism.

Chapter 8, "Positive Aging in Physical Disability and Caregiving," focuses on how positive aging can be applied to address issues of chronic disability and caregiving. Reframing these issues from a positive aging perspective involves examining what can be gained from these experiences for enhancing meaning in old age. The acknowledgment that chronic disability is inevitable, but that older persons can find quality of life and well being in its presence, is explored.

Chapter 9, "Positive Aging in Grief, Bereavement, Death, and Dying," describes issues of loss that are experienced in old age as these are captured in grief and bereavement, and addresses the psychological realities in confronting one's own death and the dying process. A positive aging approach to grief, bereavement, death, and dying is described using examples of how positive aging can aid coping as one nears the end of life.

Chapter 1

A FRAMEWORK
FOR POSITIVE AGING

THERE HAS BEEN A nearly 30-year gain in average life expectancy in the United States since 1900 when average life expectancy was 47 years (Olshansky, Carnes, & Cassel, 1990). Today, the average person can expect to live well into his or her seventh decade of life. This increase in average life expectancy means that people will not only live longer, but that population demographics will shift in favor of specific cohorts of older adults. By 2010 the U.S. Census Bureau predicts a doubling of persons 50 to 59 years of age and a 76% increase in persons 65 years and older (Kinsella & Velkoff, 2001; U.S. Centers for Disease Control, 2003). Given this backdrop it makes sense to explore ways that can enhance not only absolute human longevity, but also the qualitative aspects of how people age.

Knowing what constitutes the normative experience of human aging will likely be of interest to the lay reader seeking answers to personal questions about aging and strategies for enhancing experiences of growing older. It is also a beginning point for the practicing professional accumulating information to improve care delivery to the elderly.

NORMAL AGING

The term *normal aging*, as it appears in the scientific literature, has been closely aligned with findings from population-based longitudinal studies such as the Baltimore Longitudinal Study of Aging

(BLSA; Shock et al., 1984; Siegler, Poon, Madden, & Welsh, 1996), one of the oldest and most ambitious ongoing scientific examinations of human aging in the United States. The BLSA began in 1958, and one of its goals was to describe the normal aging experience. This included gathering data across a range of physiological, psychological, and social variables to document the nature and course of normal, or as defined by the BLSA, *nondiseased aging*. The BLSA has produced a wealth of information about normal aging, including the incontrovertible fact that (1) normal aging without disease present is different from aging when disease is present; (2) there is great heterogeneity among those people who age normally.

With respect to the relationship between diseased and nondiseased aging, in the 1980s researchers postulated that disease not only accelerates aging, but contributes to the earlier emergence of disability that, in turn, diminishes one's health and well-being (Fries, 1983; Fries & Crapo, 1981). The BLSA provided longitudinal data in support of this idea (Shock et al., 1984). These findings indicated that in the absence of disease, cardiovascular functioning in older adults was minimally affected by the aging process (Fleg & Lakatta, 1986). However, when cardiovascular function showed age-related decline, the underlying cause was almost always subthreshold coronary heart disease. In this sense, disease, not aging, was the primary culprit for cardiovascular declines associated with diminished functioning in old age. With respect to the heterogeneity of aging in BLSA participants, change in the rate of decline varied substantially across different people. In large part, interindividual differences in physiological and cognitive functioning among BLSA participants created challenges in establishing a general trajectory for age-related decline (Andres, 1985). In some cases, the interaction of aging and disease accelerated decline in function. In other cases, older persons who engaged in sustained and progressive lifestyle practices such as physical exercise, a healthy diet, and avoidance of cigarette smoking, showed minimal age-related decline in several cardiovascular indicators (Rodeheffer et al., 1984) and had equivalent functioning on some measures of health and physiological performance as sedentary younger adults.

The BLSA findings are supported by other longitudinal studies such as the Cardiovascular Health Study (CHS) that involved following nearly 3000 adults over an eight-year period. The CHS study identified persons who were aging successfully as those who were free of cardiovascular disease. They noted that although aging does eventually impact cardiovascular function, those who were free from clinical or even subclinical cardiovascular disease were able to live well into their 80s before experiencing cardiovascular deficits sufficient to produce functional decline (Newman et al., 2003).

In support of these ideas, Rowe and Kahn (1987) coined the term *normal* or *usual aging* to characterize the wide diversity in physical and cognitive function that the majority of people experience as they age. Their objective was to describe the essence of normal aging after partialing out those factors that were associated with disease. They conceptualized the inevitable consequences of growing older from middle to late adulthood, including not only from a physiological standpoint, such as the graying of one's hair, or the changing of one's body build, but also the social and psychological consequences of normal aging. The concept they espoused was simple; however, it required that age-related decline (or deterioration) be separated from disease, given that both disease and normal aging result in decline in function, but for very different reasons.

A factor that must be part of any definition of normal aging is the role of age-related decline in characterizing what it means to grow old. Although people age at different rates and in different ways, decline is a universal consequence of human aging. The specific label *normal aging*, then, can also represent an actuarial term that captures how the majority of people within a specific social or cultural group will experience decline in various functional areas. Several physiological functions are noted below as illustrative of the systemic nature of decline as it might occur in a person who is free from disease (Arking, 1998).

Heart: Maximal Volumetric Oxygen uptake declines 10% with each decade from age 25 years onward.

Lungs: Maximal lung capacity declines 40% from age 20 to 70 years.

Body Fat: Redistributes from surface to deeper parts of the body.

Muscles: Muscle mass declines 23% from 30 to 70 years.

Bones: After 35 years, bone mass declines faster than it is replaced.

These selective statistics have value for gauging how even physiological systems within a single individual are differentially affected by the rate of aging. However, as people grow older, age-related decline will vary among individuals and is dependent on a number of interrelated factors from those that are predetermined at birth (such as genetic predisposition) to those that are individually controlled or modifiable by personal lifestyle choice or environmental influence. For example, if a person begins smoking cigarettes when a teenager and continues to smoke into adulthood; even if such a person is lucky enough to avoid smoking-related diseases (such as emphysema), the rate of aging or age-related decline will likely be steeper for this person than for someone who has never smoked cigarettes.

One area that has received considerable attention in the scientific literature is the role of lifestyle choices in preserving one's physical and intellectual functioning in old age (Hubert, Bloch, Oehlert, & Fries, 2002; Hultsch, Hertzog, Small, & Dixon, 1999). It may be that there are ways that a person can act or behave in order to prevent or delay age-related decline in physical or intellectual capabilities in later life.

Warner Schaie (1994), one of the more influential researchers in adult development and aging in the 20th century studied what it meant to age normally, with a focus on intellectual change across the adult life span. Most of the information from which Schaie drew his conclusions about the aging process came from data that he examined and analyzed from the Seattle Longitudinal Study of Aging and Adult Development (SLA; Schaie, 1994, 1995, 2005). The SLA evaluated over 5000 individuals across six measurement intervals beginning in 1956 and continuing through the 1990s. The primary aim of the SLA was to explore whether there were patterns of change in intellectual functioning across adulthood that could characterize age-related decline in the normal aging population. Schaie was interested in isolating specific factors associated with the maintenance of optimal intellectual functioning in old age among persons who were otherwise disease free.

Through the research design and analysis paradigms inherent in the SLA, Schaie was able to study the nature of aging longitudinally and cross-sectionally. Thus, it was possible not only to isolate individual performance on specific measures but also assess rate of decline in any given individual participant across the SLA measurement intervals. Using this strategy, it was possible to identify specific trajectories of change in functioning with respect to how people typically grow older. In regard to intellectual abilities, most of the SLA participants showed a linear decline in intellectual functioning from their mid-40s to their 60s, especially in those abilities that were due to the neurological hardwiring of the brain or basic information processing resources that are related to the speed and efficiency with which an individual can process information. Called "fluid abilities," these include processing speed, visual peceptual dexterity, and selective aspects of short-term memory. The degradation trajectory for these abilities became markedly steeper beyond 67 years, and at this point in the aging process even abilities that one had acquired through the process of formal educational experience such as word knowledge and problem-solving skills ("crystallized abilities") were affected. This notion of age-related decline was further amplified by Giambra and his colleagues from the BLSA (Giambra, Arenberg, Zonderman, Kawas, & Costa, 1995). They also found that the mid-60s and 70s were, what they termed a *watershed period* (p. 123) for decline in intellectual functioning for both fluid and crystallized abilities. What Giambra and his colleagues meant by this notion of watershed was that at some point between the age of 65 and 75 years most people experience a precipitous diminishment in their ability to engage cognitive processes such as memory, problem solving, reasoning, and vocabulary sufficient to impair how they function on an everyday level (e.g., recalling what they saw on the news from the previous night).

Schaie, in reporting data from the SLA, found a number of other variables that influenced the rate of aging in terms of cognitive or intellectual processes including socioeconomic status, whether a person engaged in intellectually stimulating activities (such as reading, memory improvement exercises, crossword puzzles, etc.), learning memory strategies (see Chapter 3), or being married to a spouse who had high intellectual functioning. The SLA also documented that certain aspects of intellectual functioning benefited from strategic cognitive training interventions. In a subset of SLA participants who received a set of specific interventions designed to improve memory and intellectual functioning, retesting of these participants revealed that their age-related performance declines were mitigated as a consequence of this training. These findings raise the possibility that a person might be able to preserve or at least slow age-related degradation in intellectual functioning through focused training in specific intellectual skills.

Since the mid-1990s, other researchers have identified a wide range of individual difference variables to add to the list of nondisease factors that influence how a person ages (Daviglus et al., 2003; Drewnowski & Schultz, 2001; Hill, Wahlin, Winblad, & Bäckman, 1995; Reed et al., 1998). These findings, as well as results from the SLA, strongly suggest that the lifestyle choices a person makes can affect how he or she will subsequently age. In essence, we do have some control over age-related decline.

To summarize:

There is great variation in how any person ages (in the absence of disease).

Given a long enough life, everyone will eventually experience decline in physical and intellectual functioning due to aging.

An educated person who makes good lifestyle choices can, to some degree, mitigate age-related losses.

Longevity and Normal Aging

Three terms are critical for building a contemporary view of normal human aging: *average life expectancy (ALE)*, *optimum life potential (OLP)*, and *maximum life span (MLS)*.

Average life expectancy (ALE) is an actuarial average age that an individual might live given typical social conditions at a particular time. For the typical person living in the United States in 2002, the National Center for Health Statistics (2004) estimated that the ALE of an adult male at 74.5 years. The slightly greater ALE for females of 79.9 years has been speculated to be due to a combination of lifestyle and social predisposition factors, but this difference is small in comparison to one's genetic or biologically programmed maximum longevity under ideal circumstances. In the United States, ALE has been systematically lengthening for several decades. Figure 1.1 is a summary of the lengthening of ALE since 1960 for males and females of all races. Apparent in Figure 1.1 is the growth of ALE across each successive decade. For the 50-year time frame ALE has length-

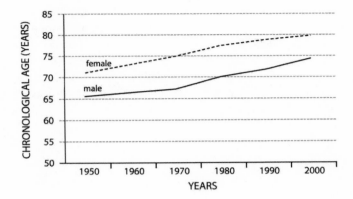

FIGURE 1.1. LIFE EXPECTANCY FROM BIRTH FOR MALES AND FEMALES. (ADAPTED FROM THE NATIONAL CENTER FOR HEALTH STATISTICS, 2004.)

ened approximately 8.7 years for males and 8.6 years for females.

Socioeconomic Factors in ALE

The economically advantaged—or those living with more resources in urban areas—versus the disadvantaged—or those in rural areas—can be distinguished by a greater ALE, which favors those with more resources or better living conditions. This is also true for those with more versus less years of formal schooling. It is likely that these as well as other demographic characteristics will become more distinguishing of optimal versus deficit aging in the 21st century and will have a profound impact on the way that normal aging is ultimately viewed both within and across social and cultural groups, especially as it relates to the number of years that a person, on average, might live. As an indication of this, Figure 1.2 contrasts black versus white, males versus females across a 50-year time interval. As can be seen from this figure, race affects ALE, with black males experiencing, on average, a shorter ALE by nearly 10 years than white females. It may be that race is an observable marker of this distinction; however, a deeper inspection reveals that black Americans in the

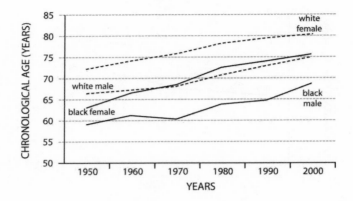

FIGURE 1.2. LIFE EXPECTANCY FROM BIRTH CONTRASTING
SEX (MALE VERSUS FEMALE) AND RACE (BLACK VERSUS
WHITE). (ADAPTED FROM THE NATIONAL CENTER FOR HEALTH
STATISTICS, 2004.)

United States, even in the present generation, tend to be in lower income stratas, less educated, and have poorer access to health care
than white Americans. And, according to these statistics, advancing
generations have not been able to narrow the ALE gap for gender
and race.

ALE as a marker of normative aging is most susceptible to changes
that occur in social and economic conditions. As the social context becomes more favorable for a specific group of persons, ALE
increases for this group and decreases for those living in less advan-
tageous circumstances. The differences in ALE between technologically advanced countries (such as the United States, Canada, and
Sweden) versus third-world countries (such as Kenya, Bangladesh,
and Afghanistan) are even more striking. The difference in ALE between these countries can be as high as 30 years in favor of those re-
gions with better living conditions.

Maximum life span (MLS) is the fixed chronological age that marks
the number of years that a member of any given species is "biologically" capable of living. At present, this is approximately 125 years
for human beings (Wilmoth, 1998). Maximum life span is the evo-
lutionary goal of every living human being, although it is rarely at-
tained, and when it is, it is likely to be due to inherent factors rather

than anything an individual did in the natural course of life. Although access to social resources may tend to increase ALE, MLS is more or less determined by characteristics intrinsic within the individual such as genetic predisposition. There are, for example, very long-lived individuals who are both rich and poor, who engage in poor versus good lifestyle behaviors, and who sometimes defy the odds with respect to disease and accidents.

There have been a number of claims of individuals who have lived up to their MLS. Take, for example, the media's reporting of the longest living person on earth, as documented through verifiable records in 1997. Her name was Jeanne Calment, and she was recorded by the *Guinness Book of Records* in 1993 as the oldest person who ever lived. Below, is an excerpt adapted from a CNN article that highlighted her longevity accomplishment as well as some of her more interesting life experiences (CNN, 1997):

> Jeanne Calment, believed to be the world's oldest person, died Monday at age 122, in Arles, France. According to her birth certificate, Calment was born on February 21, 1875. She outlived her husband, Fernand Calment, who died in 1942, four years before their 50th wedding anniversary. She also outlived her only child, a daughter who died in 1934, and her only grandson, a doctor who died in 1963. She also outlived a lawyer who hoped to take possession of her apartment. Though blind, nearly deaf, and in a wheelchair, Calment remained spirited and mentally sharp until the end. Calment credited her longevity to port wine, a diet rich in olive oil, and her sense of humor. "I will die laughing," she predicted.

Ms. Calment's story is not unlike the myriad experiences reported by the 50,000 to 70,000 centenarians who live in the United States (Kracha & Velkoff, 1999; Koplan & Fleming, 2000). A fascinating aspect of Ms. Calment's life history was that she reported being a smoker for a time, experienced poverty, and survived several diseases. From an actuarial standpoint, this would dictate a shorter ALE; however, Ms. Calment beat these odds and lived longer than any person on record.

Aging takes its toll, of course, even among these very long-living individuals, in terms of reduced stamina, decline in intellectual functioning, and the emergence of chronic physical disability. This is evident in a recently identified group of very old adults or supercentenarians, those at least 110 years of age or older, of whom it has been estimated there are between 300 and 400 worldwide. Supercentenarians, although very small in numbers, represent an important window through which the impact of age-related decline of those who are living very near the absolute MLS, can be viewed (Coles, 2004a). In a study that involved personal interviews of seven of these supercentenarians, all of whom were living in the greater Los Angeles, California area, the toll of aging was substantial (Coles, 2004a, 2004b). Unsurprisingly, all seven supercentenarians had profoundly impaired sensory function—almost all were deaf; most were blind or nearly blind; all had reduced taste and smell; all wore dentures; all had substantial muscle weakness and frailty and most were immobile; all had thin, leathery, and easily injured skin; all had poor orientation; all had compromised cognitive function, although six of the seven had fair long-term memory. These are the inevitable consequences of extreme old age or living very close to the MLS.

The third longevity term, *optimum life potential (OLP)* is, of the three terms, the most important for understanding the qualitative nature of aging. OLP is defined as the number of years that an individual, on average, should be able to live in the absence of disease, negative social conditions such as poverty or poor health care, or other external factors that could potentially shorten life. OLP is different from MLS because it includes the notion that one can influence living to one's OLP through careful lifestyle planning. At present, the OLP, as a demographic phenomenon, has been estimated to be approximately 85 years of age (Harman, 1998). Unlike MLS, OLP is an achievable aging milestone, and as more people begin living up to and beyond the OLP there will likely be significant improvements in health and quality of life for those living between the ALE and OLP. This is already emerging in a number of modern, technologically advanced societies through a process known as *the rectangularization of the survival curve* (Fries, 1983).

To understand this concept requires some familiarity with the meaning of a survival curve which, in essence, is a graphical depiction of the proportion of persons living in a specific population or group with respect to the relative age of each person in the group. As can be seen in Figure 1.3, a survival curve graphically depicts the relationship between survivability and chronological age; that is, percent surviving (Y axis) is a function of chronological age (X axis). One manifestation of this function, namely, rectangularization, indicates that greater chronological age is associated with a decreased likelihood of survival.

What is important about survival curves is the shape of the curve itself and the information that a distinctive curve provides about factors that affect aging in a given population. Figure 1.3 portrays three

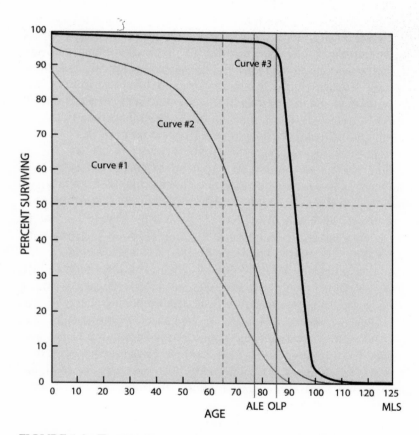

FIGURE 1.3. THREE HYPOTHETICAL SURVIVAL CURVES. (ADAPTED FROM FRIES & CRAPO, 1981.)
   ALE (Average Life Expectancy = 77 Years)
   OLP (Optimum Life Potential = 85 Years)
   MLS (Maximum Life Span = 125 Years)

hypothetical survival curves. Curve 1 takes the form of a linear trend line suggesting that the percentage of people surviving decreases uniformly with each advancing year of life. This curve shape would be typical of persons living in harsh conditions where the threat of survival is ever present from birth though adulthood. Curve 2 is slightly bulged at the midpoint, suggesting that people in this population are more likely to survive into adulthood, and it is noteworthy that the rate of dying is somewhat more confined to old age with a steeper decline after 50 years. Curve 3 follows an almost horizontal line then takes a precipitous drop in survivability after approximately 85 years, indicating a substantial death rate within a narrow age band. This drop occurs near the MLS. Curve 3 would characterize a technologically advanced population where living conditions for the majority of persons are ideal for surviving into old age. The rectangular shape of this survival curve is characteristic of optimal survival followed by a compression of morbidity into the latter end of the life span (Fries, 1981; Fries & Crapo, 1981).

Based on this concept, Fries (1980; see also Fries, 1983; Fries & Crapo, 1981) argued that as ALE approaches OLP, for the larger percentage of older persons, morbidity would be compressed into a narrow age range between OLP and MLS. This hypothetical relationship can be seen in Figure 1.3 where OLP and MLS represent a kind of confidence interval within which death occurs (Curve 3). The public health implications of a rectangularized survival function are that increased longevity should also produce better quality of life as well. In fact, several studies have documented that as people live longer they find ways to live healthier lives. Healthy living, in this regard, is achieved not only through improved medical technologies, but also by making lifestyle choices that maximize optimal health and longevity including: better diet, exercise, avoiding harmful substances such as heavy alcohol drinking, illicit drug use, and smoking, as well as disease prevention efforts that are associated with longevity, including regular diagnostic health examinations (i.e., mamographies, colonoscopies) and controlling diagnosed medical conditions such as high cholesterol and high blood pressure (Hubert, Bloch, Oehlert, & Fries, 2002).

Evidence has begun to accumulate that validates this claim. Dutch researchers, for example, put the rectangularization hypothesis to the test on historical demographic data, available to them from Dutch government records, of morbidity rates from 1950 to 1992 (Nusselder, Mackenbach, & Mackenbach, 1996). They restricted this data to those persons who were 60 years and older and found that with each progressive generation, the pattern of morbidity began to compress near the MLS. The survival function was rectangularizing in this society. If replicated in other first world countries (such as Sweden, the United States, and Germany), the implications of this pattern of longevity, in terms of improved quality of life, could have a substantial impact on how health care and aging will be viewed in the 21st century. Fries (1980 & 1983; see also Fries & Crapo, 1981) predicted that as fewer persons in these countries languish in poor health in their 70s and 80s, the demand for long-term care for the elderly would be somewhat attenuated. Although an intuitively appealing notion, this latter postulate has yet to be empirically confirmed.

It is important to underscore that there are a number of requirements that are essential for such a rectangularization function to occur in a social system. The majority of members of a society must engage in preventive health behaviors and be relatively free from chronic disease earlier in life. For these individuals, a good quality of life would be an expectation of living into one's eighth decade, with a relatively rapid decline in health and functioning once a person exceeded the actuarial OLP, as noted earlier. The exceptions to this rule would be those persons who adopted poor lifestyle habits early in life such as chronic smoking, overeating, and a sedentary lifestyle, or those who had chronic disease or an accident at an earlier point in the life span in childhood or adulthood. A person's lifestyle choices would impact, in a significant way, not only the quality of old age, but absolute longevity as well.

SUCCESSFUL AGING

The term *successful aging* was popularized by Rowe and Kahn (1998) to describe those older individuals who are able to live beyond the ALE and experience quality aging into the seventh and eighth decades of life. What is of interest in this regard are the lifestyle behaviors that characterize successful agers and the extent to which those behaviors can be adopted by others in the 21st century as a way to live into very old age.

Descriptions of *successful aging* have appeared in the scientific literature for more than five decades. In the 1950s the term described a person's ability to optimally adapt to old age (Baker, 1958). As a term that explained a qualitatively unique process inherent in increased longevity, one of the earliest definitions of successful aging was proposed by Havighurst (1961) who labeled *successful agers* as those persons who: (1) lived longer with respect to number of years or absolute longevity and (2) could find life satisfaction in later life. In 1982, Ryff, in a similar vein, characterized successful aging as an idealized form of human functioning that resulted in optimal adult development across the lifespan. In *The Encyclopedia of Aging*, Palmore (1995) provided one of the more comprehensive definitions of successful aging as a combination of optimal survival capability, health, and the experience of life satisfaction in old age.

Optimal aging has been described as a variant of successful aging (Hill et al., 1995). However, the term *optimal aging* was construed to represent a more restricted form of aging based on inherent biological and/or genetic characteristics of the individual that work to maximize longevity. In one study, Hill et al. (1995) found that a small group of optimally aging older Swedish adults from the Kungsholmen Project, which is a longitudinal population-based study on aging and dementia that is ongoing in Stockholm, Sweden, showed minimal cognitive decline on measures of verbal and fluid abilities into the eighth decade of life.

Rowe and Kahn (1987) suggested that successful aging is represented by individuals who experience little or no age-related decline, even though they might be living into the seventh or eighth decade of life. They asserted that successful agers were a category of persons who were living a lifestyle that promoted quality aging up to, and in some instances beyond, the established OLP. These persons, by virtue of their inherent physiological constitution, pro-health lifestyle choices, and personal disposition, managed to minimize age-related decline in as much as they experienced fewer deficits in physical or mental functioning than the general population of older adults. Rowe and Kahn defined successful aging as: low risk of disease and disease-related disability; high mental and physical function; and active engagement in life.

Using this definition, successful aging was operationalized as a process of growing old that was resistant to the deteriorative forces of aging. Thus, individuals identified as successful agers were, in a sense, "entitled" to experience, as a consequence of positive lifestyle choices and behaviors, happiness, fulfillment, and good health in old and very old age.

In addition to the notion of successful aging, an underlying assumption was that persons who were successful agers would have a history of facilitative developmental experiences in earlier life (e.g., a good education, access to high-quality health care) including learning "how" to make positive lifestyle choices (such as regular exercise) to enhance their ability to maintain a high degree of well-being and life satisfaction in old age. Successful aging presumes that there are specific activities that a person could engage in that would make it possible to live up to (or beyond) the OLP.

The MacArthur Studies of Successful Aging was initiated in 1984, with the goal of identifying a cohort of high-functioning successful agers between 70 and 79 drawn from three communities: Durham, NC, East Boston, MA, and New Haven, CT. Study participants were administered an extensive battery of tests to assess physical performance, cognitive functioning, health status, and psychological characteristics and capabilities. These measures were taken over multiple time periods in order to examine and track the extent to which age-related change could be documented from these markers of functionality (Seeman, et al, 1994; Tabbarah, Crimmins & Seeman, 2002).

Findings from the MacArthur Studies of Successful Aging are well known in the scientific literature (Benkman et al., 1995; Rowe & Kahn, 1998) and they confirm several of the assumptions made about successful aging: There are individuals who appear to age optimally; there are specific characteristics about a person that produce successful aging; there are activities and lifestyle choices that facilitate successful aging; even in successful aging, age-related decline is still present (Seeman et al., 1994).

Successful aging is an important term, then, not only for understanding that aging can have positive consequences, but that it is possible to engage in behaviors in adulthood that will make a difference in how a person ages. People are to some extent in charge and responsible for their own quality of life in old age.

Even though *successful aging* is an idealized term that, at present, does not reflect the nature of aging for most people in our society, it is a useful concept and informative about normative processes of growing old. A successful ager would be a nonsmoker, for example, and a consequence of not smoking could be not only greater longevity but a better quality of life overall. *Successful aging* was one of the first terms to acknowledge that a person can act in ways to make his or her life better in old and very old age.

POSITIVE AGING

The backdrop for positive aging can be found in Seligman and Csikszentmihalyi's work on positive psychology (Seligman & Csikzentmihalyi, 2000). Among the many features of positive psychology that are useful for understanding positive aging is the premise that human beings possess strengths and resources that can buffer them against challenges that they might encounter across the life span. Seligman names specific strengths as follows: "courage, future mindedness, optimism, interpersonal skill, faith, work ethic, hope, honesty, perseverance, and the capacity for flow and insight. . ." (p. 7).

The term *positive aging* describes an individual acting on the resources available to her or him to optimize the aging experience; that is, in Seligman's terms (Seligman & Csikszentmihalyi, 2000), positive aging makes the process of growing old a worthwhile experience. These resources include psychological factors that are intrinsic but are, for the most part, amenable to one's will or state of mind (e.g., courage), the environment (e.g., medical care practices, housing, occupation, etc.), as well as individual traits such as personality, values, attitudes, and beliefs that tend to be stable across the life span but that can also be accessed as a source of coping with the aging process. Unlike terms such as *senility, decrepitude, degeneration,* and *infirmity* that are used to categorize older persons into groups that represent loss or decay, positive aging makes several new assumptions about old age and events that can be anticipated to occur in late life. The most central of these is the assumption that it is possible to modify one's own aging experience.

This notion of positive aging as a term descriptive of a person acting on his or her environment to enhance the quality of living in later life regardless of the deficits or emotional liabilities that one may have encountered in the past was alluded to by George Valliant in the final chapter of his book, *Aging Well* (Valliant, 2002). He observes that, "Positive aging must always reflect vital reaction to change, to disease, and to environmental imbalance. Positive aging is not simply avoidance of physical decay, and it certainly is not avoidance of death (p. 161)." Actively shaping the aging process involves more than finding ways to evade the negative consequences of growing old, but involves recognizing that decline, loss, and even one's own death are natural parts of the life cycle, and that it is possible to shape how one interprets these events. The concept of positive aging does not ignore the realities of old age but instead, focuses on the idea that there are actions one can take to enhance well-being, even in the presence of age-related decline and loss. The point here is that choice makes a difference, even in the most difficult aging scenarios.

To get a more concrete picture of the nature and scope of positive aging it may be possible to characterize it with respect to specific lifestyle choices. There are many types of behaviors that can result in reduced longevity; take, for example, cigarette smoking. With respect to positive aging, the focus is less on how cigarette smoking may shorten length of life, but how long a person will enjoy well-being (or quality of life) in old age while continuing to smoke. Cigarette smoking is a lifestyle choice that may not only reduce absolute longevity, but may also interact with the deteriorative processes of aging and speed age-related decline (Hill, Nilsson, Nyberg, & Bäckman, 2003). Chronic smoking is incompatible with positive aging and quitting cigarette smoking would be a lifestyle choice that affirms a positive aging lifestyle. This is also true of a myriad of lifestyle behaviors including overeating, the avoidance of physical exercise, failure to wear a seatbelt while driving, engaging in destructive behaviors such as excessive gambling, overspending, illicit drug use, or abusing alcohol or prescription medications. Positive aging requires some discipline, but the consequences are greater well-being and better adaptation in later life (Wister, 2003).

Characteristics of Positive Aging

The question that arises is whether there are characteristics that would be indicative of positive aging and if it is possible to cultivate positive aging as a way to not only optimize a longer life span, but

17

also better quality of life in the process. What follows are four characteristics of of positive aging.

First Positive Aging Characteristic: A Person Mobilizes Resources to Cope with Age-related Decline

A person deals with age-related decline by mobilizing the necessary resources to remain satisfied with life even in the course of decline. This is because age-related decline and positive aging are not mutually exclusive. There is a 50% chance that a person who lives to be 85 years of age or older will experience at least one age-related disability (Manton, Corder, & Stallard, 1997). Given this scenario, it would be consistent with a positive aging perspective to acknowledge that disability is an inevitable outcome of age-related decline, to be planned for with respect to gauging how one will cope with it. Two types of coping that an older person might engage in to preserve his or her quality of life, even in the presence of age-related decline, have been described by Brandstedter (1990). He suggested two types: (1) *Assimilative coping* or the acknowledgment that in order to achieve a desired objective that has become unobtainable due to age-related decline one must approach the task in a new way. For example, if one's vision deteriorates to the point where even with glasses it is difficult to read the newspaper, assimilative coping would involve purchasing a magnifying lens in order to offset poor vision. (2) *Accommodative coping* when progressive disability makes a desired goal unobtainable, such as when vision loss makes reading a newspaper no longer possible even with aids. This involves permanently altering one's preferences or attitudes about a desired goal or objective that is no longer possible to achieve. For example, the older person with vision loss who can no longer read a newspaper may change his or her own preferences from reading newsprint to listening to the radio or, he or she may simply decide that current events are no longer of interest. These two coping strategies have been found to offset negative emotional reactions to loss, including hopelessness or depression, that are commonly experienced by the elderly (Blazer, 2003). They often occur in conjunction with one another; that is, an older person may shift from an assimilative form of coping, when a capability is impaired but still intact, to accommodative coping when he or she can no longer perform the particular task (Boerner, 2004).

It can sometimes be the case, particularly in institutional care contexts, that accommodative coping is used even when an older patient or client still has the physical and psychological resources to address a disability with an assimilative coping response. In a unique naturalistic study that examined the well-being of older persons who were residing in a nursing home, when staff did not attend to a patient's capabilities to perform a task, and, as a consequence, provided only an accommodative coping option, the well-being and life satisfaction of the resident suffered (Kayser-Jones, 2002). For example, the tendency of the staff to diaper all older residents for incontinence, even those who were still able to toilet themselves, was viewed as not only unhelpful and demeaning, but also as sending the message that there was little encouragement for residents to maintain their dignity in independent functioning. It is important for mental health professionals who are working with older clients, whether in an inpatient or outpatient setting, to not only understand the dynamics of coping in old age but to identify strategies that optimize a client's unique capabilities to deal with an age-related disability in order to preserve functioning and quality of life.

Second Positive Aging Characteristic: A Person Makes Lifestyle Choices to Preserve Well-being

A person makes lifestyle choices that emphasize the preservation of psychological and physical resources. The German Aging Survey, a longitudinal investigation that began in 1996 (Steverink, Westerhof, Bode, & Dittmann-Kohli, 2001) examined the personal perceptions of adults ages 40 to 85. Three themes emerged that defined, for the study participants, what was important with respect to their view of old age, and what was critical to invest effort into preserving: (1) Issues of physical decline (health and vitality)—the important feature here was to preserve functioning by minimizing age-related decline as much as possible. (2) Growth and personal development—the importance of lifelong learning was underscored. For most people, in sickness or in health, quality of life is integrally connected to the need to develop oneself personally throughout the life span. (3) Loss of others in the social network—in old age, the importance of lifelong relationships and the preservation of relationships are central to well-being.

These three themes provide a taxonomy of what is important in preserving well-being in old age. For example, the first area, health and its preservation, is an important theme that is a life span issue and it is no less important in youth and adulthood than it is in old age. For this reason, discovering ways to maintain (or improve) one's health in old age is essential. Even if a person is declining it should not be a barrier to seeking out ways to optimize health in other areas of functioning (Furstenberg, 2002). For example, people in their 40s might develop a plan to engage in preventive health behaviors such as eating a more balanced diet or beginning an exercise program to preserve health for as long as possible. For those who are 80 years old, however, the issue of health maintenance may take a somewhat different form, such as scheduling more frequent visits to the health clinic for specialized health checkups in order to better assess the progression of a chronic illness. It might also take the form of making decisions about which activities one can still participate in versus those that should be avoided. For example, an older person may decide to adjust a lifelong pattern of running as a form of exercise given the emergence of knee and back problems, and to replace this activity with brisk walking in order to preserve the health benefits of such activity without causing undue physical stress on declining knee and back functioning.

The second area, finding meaningful ways to engender personal growth experiences, would suggest that finding new learning opportunities or creating avenues in which one can continue to learn, would be critical in preserving positive aging. The effort to find ways to engage in lifelong learning can, in and of itself be an enrichment opportunity. In youth, formal education is not only a social expectation, but it is a clear roadmap for ongoing intellectual development. The same kinds of resources are available for the older adult as well, although it may require that the older person engage in a search for educational experiences that fit her or his own personal learning style and disposition for self-development.

The third area would suggest that it is important to develop strategies for dealing with the inevitability of losing loved ones (such as a spouse) to death or the consequences of a chronic disease such as Alzheimer's. Positive agers learn what is meaningful to them and then prioritize strategies that they can engage to remediate, preserve, or even enhance those sources of meaning. Sources of meaning are not the same for every person; however, the themes noted above are important to consider if one desires to optimize well-being and satisfaction in old age.

Third Positive Aging Characteristic: A Person Cultivates Flexibility Across the Life Span

The concept of flexibility has been defined in the psychological literature as a person's capacity to invoke novel strategies of behaving or thinking to promote better problem solving and/or adaptation. From an intellectual framework, Schaie (2005) defined flexibility as an approach to cognitive problem solving that involved the dynamic manipulation of multiple solution sets to yield the best outcome in the shortest amount of time. Flexibility as a psychological coping mechanism involves the balancing of one's existing skills and personal resources to optimize adaptation to psychological stressors (Lazarus & Folkman, 1984). Flexibility, therefore, represents a central characteristic of positive aging. Rozanski & Kubzansky (2005) identified specific behaviors that were indicative of emotional and coping flexibility including "adjusting goals or priorities to cope with changing circumstances, setting limits, invoking social support, and seeking advice or counseling" (p. 50). In addition, they hypothesized that persons who were better able to flexibly regulate their emotional responses to stressors should be better protected from disease and emotional illness (Bonanno, Papa, O'Neil, Westphal, & Coifman, 2004). Flexibility, then, is an important marker of positive aging that suggests a person can create meaning and optimism in the presence of physical or psychological decline.

The scientific literature also suggests that flexibility is a skill that one can acquire through strategic practice and effort (Cheng, 2001). Activities that promote flexibility are those that connect an older person to her or his deepest sources of personal meaning. Approaches to living that tend to require flexibility include the capacity to forgive others (and even oneself) for injustices and/or failures in life, the ability to shape personal goals to optimize well-being in the face of the realities of age-related decline, and the capacity to engage in generative acts that serve to enhance the best interests of others, even if this is at the expense of not meeting some self-needs. These examples of flexibility are described in more detail in Chapter 7. At this juncture, however, it is important to highlight the general concept of flexibility, its

21

consequences, and its role as a pivotal positive aging characteristic. The underlying assumption is that flexibility, like the other positive aging characteristics described earlier, can be learned over the course of living and through coping with life's challenges.

Fourth Positive Aging Characteristic: A Person Focuses on the Positives versus the Problems and Difficulties of Growing Old

People sometimes focus on the negative aspects of aging. In a national survey that queried whether older adults would be willing to consider nursing home placement, 30% of the respondents acknowledged that they would rather die than be placed in a nursing home (Mattimore et al., 1997). When an individual experiences this level of pessimistic anticipation, the act of planning for the future can be a daunting task. So, understandably, some people simply ignore their own aging to avoid these unpleasant inevitabilities (the diagnosis of osteoarthritis, the diminishment of one's eyesight). While it is true that those who live into old and very old age will experience age-related decline, including disability, perhaps assisted living or nursing home placement and eventually death, these life span challenges do not preclude cultivating a positive attitude in the present toward one's own aging experience. In fact, research suggests that well-being and life satisfaction are, in many respects, relative emotional states independent of one's objective health, living situation, or socioeconomic standing (Diener, 2000 Diener & Diener, 1996). Positive aging, therefore, may represent a state of mind that is more than a static appraisal of one's own objective condition, but a cultivated sense of well-being that can come from optimistically appraising one's sense of integrity in spite of declining faculties. Some people are better at this than others. Research studies have affirmed that cultivating a positive attitude by focusing selectively on the meaningful aspects of one's old age (i.e., the care received from family members, living to see future generations) can be a robust source of personal satisfaction (Freund, Alexandra, & Baltes, 1998; Fredrickson, 2000). The ability to generate a positive sense of well-being, even in difficult times, can take many forms including gratitude, counting one's blessings, and thankfulness or thanksgiving for the positives that one experiences (Emmons & McCullough, 2004). George Valliant in his book, *Aging Well* (2002) provides examples of individuals who made the conscious choice to focus on the positive meaning of age-related decline and the role that this way of thinking plays in promoting a sense of well-being and life satisfaction in old and very old age. Valliant also reported that the cultivation of an optimistic attitude toward one's old age was not confined to those who were well educated and wealthy, but was also present in several older study participants who were living in poverty and had very little formal education.

In a sense, these four characteristics reflect what George Valliant meant by this notion of positive aging as a form of "aging well" (Valliant, 2002).

CONCLUDING COMMENTS

This chapter explores various terms that characterize the aging experience. Different types of aging were defined: *normal aging, successful aging,* and *positive aging.* The unique features of positive aging were described along with some specific characteristic that can facilitate the positive aging experience. Because positive aging is essentially a psychological construct or a state of mind, it is obtainable either in the presence of health or in illness. It does, however, require deliberate effort to engage a positive aging mindset, and, for this reason, describing how to cultivate positive aging while coping with the personal challenges of growing old is an essential goal of this book.

Chapter 2

THREE LIFE SPAN MODELS
OF AGING

THREE MODELS OF ADULT human development are summarized in this chapter: Erikson's stage theory of life span development (Erikson 1963, 1980); continuity theory (Atchley, 1989); and selectivity, optimization, and compensation (SOC) theory (Baltes, 1997). The link between these models and positive aging is highlighted and a case example is presented that demonstrates how these theoretical constructs can be applied within a counseling intervention that employs positive aging to address an age-specific issue.

ERIKSON'S STAGES OF ADULT DEVELOPMENT

Erikson was one of the first scholars of adult human development to recognize the manifestations of maturation as an outcome of developmental processes (Friedman, 1999). Maturation, in Erikson's view, was the successful resolution of predictable age-graded crises as these unfolded across the life span (1980). Erikson, unlike Freud who viewed developmental processes as only occurring during childhood and adolescence (Freud, 1905/1953), saw maturation as an ongoing process in adulthood and believed that adults continued to mature as they worked to resolve developmental crises throughout the life span. For Erikson, the consequence of mastering each life stage was the acquisition of a specific aspect of maturity; namely, hope, will, purpose, competence, fidelity, love, caring, and wisdom (Erikson, Erikson, & Kivnick, 1986). These stages of adult development are described in Figure 2.1, a widely published schematic of Erikson's eight stages of life. The satisfactory resolution of each stage produces, as a consequence, a specific life outlook or worldview that is a manifestation of maturity.

STAGE	Basic Trust & Basic Mistrust HOPE	Autonomy & Shame/Doubt WILL	Initiative & Guilt PURPOSE	Industry & Inferiority COMPETENCE	Identity & Confusion FIDELITY	Intimacy & Isolation LOVE	Generativity & Self-absorption CARE	Integrity & Despair WISDOM
AGE	Birth to 1	2 to 3	4 to 5	6 to 12	13 to 19	20 to 45	45 to 65	70+

FIGURE 2.1. ERIKSON'S LIFE SPAN DEVELOPMENT. (ADAPTED FROM *VITAL INVOLVEMENT IN OLD AGE*, BY E. H. ERIKSON AND H. Q. KIVNICK, 1986. NEW YORK: W. W. NORTON. COPYRIGHT © 1986 BY W. W. NORTON & CO.)

Trust vs. Mistrust

This stage is encountered from birth to age 12 months as the infant forms an attachment with his or her primary caregiver (typically the mother). In order for the infant's basic needs to be met, the caregiver must be trusted. Problems arise if the caregiver is rejecting or inconsistent. Under these circumstances, the infant may not develop a basic sense of trust. Instead, he or she may view the world as a dangerous place filled with unreliable people. Successfully negotiating this crisis results in a positive outlook of the future that is not stifled by fear. Such a worldview can then facilitate the development of meaningful future social relationships. The specific form of maturity that emerges from the resolution of this first stage is *hope*, defined as a feeling that what one wants in the future will transpire. Hope is the foundation of optimism, one of the basic building blocks of positive aging.

Autonomy vs. Shame and Doubt

This stage is encountered from approximately age 2 to 3 years when the child is confronted with the need to become independent in negotiating activities of daily living. The critical task here is that the child must learn to feed and dress her- or himself, including

25

taking responsibility for maintaining self-care behaviors. In many cases these are not difficult skills to acquire; however, challenges arise if the child is prevented from learning to independently engage in these activities or to develop autonomy. Self-sufficiency occurs when the child exercises his or her will as an independent person. In this situation if the child's efforts to become autonomous are rebuffed he or she may develop self-doubt, and come to view the world as a difficult place where one's determination might be overpowered by others. The form of maturity that emerges from this developmental stage is the belief that through the exercise of one's own *will* it is possible to achieve one's goals and aspirations in life.

Initiative vs. Guilt

This stage is encountered from approximately 4 to 5 years of age when the child attempts more difficult tasks that challenge his or her capacities. It is critical to undertake responsibilities or life tasks that require not only effort and will, but initiative as well. In some cases this initiative may conflict with the wishes of important others, including parents and other family members. Resolution of this stage involves retaining one's sense of initiative while at the same time learning not to interfere with the values or rights of others. If this stage is not successfully negotiated, the negative consequence is a sense of guilt, particularly when the child engages in future activities that are seen as conflicting with the family's value system. This stage is critical to the development of values and ideals. Most important for life span development, successfully negotiating this stage results in a form of maturity that affirms *purpose* in living.

Industry vs. Inferiority

This stage is encountered from approximately 6 to 13 years of age, or puberty, when the child is confronted with the need to learn the skills necessary for managing her- or himself in a complex world. The child must acquire important social, physical, and academic skills. This is a period when the child tends to compare him- or herself to peers. This comparison often leads to a sense that one needs to work hard in order to keep up with one's own peer group. By successfully competing with his or her own peers, the child acquires the everyday skills that are the basis of self-reliance, which are needed to move through adolescence. Failure to acquire these important attributes leads to feelings of inferiority and self-doubt. The form of maturity developed by successfully negotiating this life stage is a sense of *competence*.

Identity vs. Confusion

This stage is encountered in adolescence and young adulthood (from approximately 13 to 19 years) and is, perhaps, the best known of Erikson's stages. The critical juncture here is to learn to act independently, balanced by the fact that there are objective constraints to independent living embedded in social rules and traditions. It is for this reason that the behaviors often associated with this stage take the form of rebellion against parents, teachers, and society (Erikson, 1968). Reconciliation with social norms, however, is one of the critical issues within this stage that leads to health and well-being. Identity versus role confusion, then, represents the first stage of Erikson's developmental model that is demonstrative of adult socialization. It is negotiation of this stage that characterizes the fully functioning adult. The form of maturity that emerges from negotiating this developmental stage is *fidelity*, or faithful devotion to social values, to others, and to oneself.

Intimacy vs. Isolation

This stage is encountered during the course of adulthood (from approximately 20 to 40+ years) and has a particularly long duration. Those who are able to negotiate the predictable tasks of adulthood are better able to develop and sustain meaningful relationships across the life course. It is important at this stage to form friendships that are lasting and to achieve a sense of love and companionship with others. Feelings of loneliness or isolation are the consequences of one's inability to form friendships or intimate relationships during this period. Romantic companions, spouses, and close friends represent the affiliations that are critical for the maturing adult at this stage of development. The successful resolution of this stage is the ability to feel genuine *love* for others.

Generativity vs. Self-Absorption

This stage is encountered in what could be termed one's entry into middle adulthood (from approximately 46 to 55 years of age). During this period the adult faces the task of becoming productive in his or her job or career and in caring for the needs of younger, more vulnerable people. This stage focuses on how the individual is able to function purposefully within his or her own culture. Those who are unable to assume these responsibilities tend to be self-centered. However, those individuals who are able to negotiate this life stage develop empathy for others. A critical behavior that characterizes this stage is assisting the younger generation to develop into purposeful adults. When a person is not able to negotiate this stage, a feeling of impotence emerges. A person may sincerely believe that he or she has done nothing to help the next generation. This feeling was characterized by Erikson as emotional stagnation. The form of maturity that emerges from successfully negotiating this stage is the ability to care for others.

Integrity vs. Despair

This stage is encountered in what is characterized as old age (from approximately 60 years to the end of life). During this stage the mature adult looks back on one's own life with the goal of evaluating its meaning or purpose. In this regard, life is viewed along a values-based continuum as either being productive and happy or disappointing. Life span experiences, particularly social experiences, often determine the outcome of this final life stage. *Wisdom* emerges from the successful negotiation of this stage. A wise person understands that the future, near the end of life, will ultimately take care of itself and is not worth worrying about. Thus, for the person who negotiates this stage successfully, fear of death is replaced by peace of mind and a sense of appreciation for a life well lived.

ERIKSON'S THEORY AND POSITIVE AGING

Can Erikson's eight life stages be linked to the concept of positive aging? To answer this question one must understand three basic premises of adult development: (1) internal forces inherent within the individual from birth create pressures on the individual to evolve, change, and mature; (2) external forces in the social world acting on the individual influence how a person feels and behaves; (3) these two forces interact to shape the individual from birth to death.

In relation to Erikson's scheme of psychosocial development, positive aging is the ability to understand that one's own personal needs, at times, should be subordinated in order to promote the larger good of others. Early in life this subordination is to the mother, then the family, then one's peer group, then the extended family and the community. This reasoning underscores the point that there is a personal dynamic and a specific reference group that must be involved in the negotiation and resolution of each of Erikson's life stages of development. Resolving predictable crises at each stage in the life course will likely result in optimal development, and will produce emotional capacities that are essential to positive aging, such as hope, will, purpose in life, competence, fidelity, love, caring, and wisdom.

Erikson's theory implies that the eight stages of development occur in evenly spaced intervals across the life span and that the progression toward maturity moves forward from each stage to the next. However, to place these complex human emotions along a linear continuum runs the risk of oversimplifying what it means to mature as an adult and how a person engages in positive aging as a developmental skill in this process. Recent evidence suggests that the encountering and resolving of each of these life stages may occur at different times for different persons (Kowaz & Marcia, 1991). In fact, some research indicates that many of the maturational milestones Erikson described as occurring in childhood are, in fact, negotiated by some people in early and middle adulthood, and it is possible that a person might revisit, in later life, earlier stages of development that were unresolved (Whitbourne & Waterman, 1979; Whitbourne, Zuschlag, Elliot, & Waterman, 1992).

Whether there are certain time periods that are more amenable to resolving a particular developmental crisis than others remains an open question. However, what appears to be supported by research is that people do change with respect to maturity in old age just as they do in youth and childhood (Whitbourne & Waterman, 1979; Whitbourne et al., 1992). The circumstances that catalyze developmental change may be quite different for younger versus older adults, however. For example, in old age, the loss of one's job may have a profound effect on maturational processes related to "competence," even more than a loss that may have occurred earlier in adulthood. Further, a person who lacks a sense of "competence" may be able to develop this maturational characteristic through counseling and education. Positive agers are people who continue to improve their own sense of self in later life by engaging strategies designed to build maturity.

Issues in Application

Mary, a 77-year-old widow, lived alone in her home and reported feeling lonely and despondent on most days. She described her life as being filled with missed opportunities. When pressed, she was quick to attribute many of her problems to an unhappy childhood with parents who never put forth much effort to help her through several difficult childhood transitions, "My mother's controlling behaviors have lived in my memories ever since I was 4 years old and I have a vivid memory of those days. . . ." It was these memories that Mary believed led her to make a very poor decision to marry the "wrong" man, and then to suffer with this difficult husband for 50 years only to have the marriage end when he died of emphysema. Mary explained, "I wanted to have my own career before I was married." Although Mary had two children who regularly visited her, she was reluctant to talk about them in any detail. For Mary, her complaining focused mainly on her own experiences, her poor marriage, and her resentment that she was prevented from pursuing a career for herself.

Mary's case is relevant to Erikson's theory of adult development, first, because she clearly reported experiencing a difficult childhood (whether real or imagined) that left her with a number of maladaptive tendencies. One of these was a worldview of disappointment underlying a perceived inability to realize her own dreams. In some sense, Mary seemed to lack the capacity for developing her own purpose and direction in life. Mary's negative feelings about being disappointed many times during the course of her life left her with a poor sense of the purpose for her existence. Mary's current tendency was to engage in wishful thinking about how her life might have been better had these negative life experiences been different. At age 77, she was developmentally frozen due to her focused view of these early negative events that had made it difficult for her to find peace of mind in her later years. Mary seemed unable to find meaning in life. This was the case even when there were potential sources of meaning for her including her children and the role that she might play in their lives.

Lost causes, missed opportunities, and negative life experiences are part of every life lived; however, old age need not be entirely stifled by these if one can find a positive perspective upon which to reflect. In Mary's case, what she desperately needed was to feel that her life had a sense of purpose. If one were to take a more detailed history from Mary, it is likely that she lacked the initiative to find purpose in a number of aspects of her daily life even before she began thinking about a career for herself. If she acted on a sense of purpose, it was with the short-term goal of escaping something that she perceived was difficult (e.g., marrying young to escape from home). When she faced the challenges inherent in the life stage (initiative vs. guilt) she was likely unable to resolve this in a way that would allow her to mature. This was not entirely due to her own internal processes, but involved a complex interaction of the social world that she lived in, family pressures, and her own capacities for change and personal growth over the course of her life span.

What was important for the present, however, was to help Mary find a sense of purpose in her life. Could she somehow return to an early stage of development and then work to resolve this even though she was 77 years old?

The answer to this question is both yes and no. The process by which this could occur would be difficult for her and would likely have required reconstrual of her past memories. Therefore, the steps to finding positive aging for Mary are highlighted below and are illustrative of how Erikson's life stage model might be a useful guide for counseling or psychotherapy:

1. Identify where Mary was, in the present, with respect to Erikson's developmental stages and what may have occurred in the past that was preventing her from negotiating the present stage. In Mary's case the stage consistent with her chronological age-graded crisis was integrity vs. despair. As was noted

above, the task for this stage is the engagement of a reflective life span review. Mary is unable to engage this process partly because of her own lack of purpose and lack of meaning in her life.

2. Identify an earlier stage where there was some evidence that Mary has had difficulty resolving issues. The marker for this would be Mary's inability to engage in the mature behavior that would characterize the resolution of a specific life stage. In this case, Mary was unable to articulate a sense of purpose.

3. Help Mary rediscover a sense of purpose. Although she had much to complain about, including her view that life had been unfair, there may be more constructive memories that she could choose to recollect. In this regard, a counselor might encourage Mary to focus on describing those events across the course of her life that helped her find a sense of purpose in living. This may be difficult, at first, given Mary's practiced pattern of negative construal of her earlier life experiences; however, it would be important for her to begin such a process in order to find alternative sources of fulfillment. Mary might be encouraged to think about her children and the value that she represents to them. This strategy would necessarily involve avoiding the futility of trying to "change" the past, as well as the activity of anticipating the future. However, her children could be a source of meaning or purpose in her life.

4. Over the course of time and with professional help, Mary could learn to acknowledge a purpose for living and begin to think in a somewhat different way about herself. She could be a source of well-being and support for others, including her children. This might involve trying to cultivate renewed relationships with those who are around her including her family and friends. Through these relationships, finding a more enduring sense of the present could be possible.

Within the Eriksonian model of adult development, childhood experiences are emphasized as precursors to the development of problem-solving skills in adulthood. In Mary's case, many of her articulated disappointments occurred in the past and she had a vivid memory of those events in childhood. Unfortunately, as is often the case in old age, those persons involved in the negative events may no longer be living. So, it is simply not possible to alter these relationships or circumstances in any real way. Further, it may be that earlier events are lost from memory. If this is the case, then resolving such forgotten issues would be irrelevant for promoting well-being.

It would be possible in Mary's case, however, to help her begin to rediscover a sense of purpose by reconstructing those early memories with the goal of finding new meanings within them. Finding alternative ways to construe events can be a powerful way to foster well-being from an otherwise painful past. The ability to reframe negative memories in order to make them more manageable to live with is at the basis of a positive aging lifestyle. It may also be possible to simply let go of negative memories in the past by focusing on present circumstances. It might be that Mary could let go of her past by focusing on the degree to which her living children are currently interested in her. She might want to find out what sustains that interest. Likely, it will be something in the present as opposed to a memory from the past.

The strength of Erikson's approach is its rich description of the stages a person will encounter (and need to negotiate) as one grows older. If it is the case that people can resolve developmental crises and continue to mature across the life span, then it represents a number of opportunities for interventions designed to enhance or build maturation processes in old age. The next two theories—continuity theory and SOC—provide the basis for developing intervention strategies to help older adults address the challenges of living. These theories are, for the most part, rooted in adulthood and old age. Aside from some minor allusions to childhood, it is the adult experience of living that shapes how a person finds positive aging in later life.

CONTINUITY THEORY

Continuity theory is a social–psychological theory of aging based on the premise that one's identity in old age is influenced by one's enduring self-perceptions and the contextual factors that influence the stability of this self-view. Robert Atchley (1989) proposed the term *continuity theory* to describe the role that consistency, or a lack thereof, plays in defining one's sense of self as an "older person." He argued that the personal experience of aging is influenced by two sources of consistency that he labeled *internal continuity* and *external continuity*. Atchley notes: "in making adaptive choices, middle-aged and older adults attempt to preserve and maintain existing internal and external structures . . . as a primary adaptive strategy for dealing with normal aging" (1989, p. 193).

Continuity theory also considers the role of change in shaping one's sense of self. Change, from a continuity point of view, involves two processes, first the small increments of maturation that occur within the individual with the passage of time; second, more dramatic shifts in the individual or in his or her context. These large changes he labeled as *discontinuities* and they can be interpreted as either positive (winning the lottery) or negative (death of a loved one), but they always involve an initial disruption in one's external world or a challenge to one's inner self.

Internal Continuity

Internal continuity is the sense of oneself in the present that is, in part, a reflection of self-identity in the past. The basis of internal continuity is that there are stable internal personal characteristics that tend to dictate how adaptable a person might be in old age and the extent to which change is possible for a given individual. The vignette below is an example of internal continuity:

John, age 55, was the controller of a small but profitable construction firm, which had been purchased by a large multinational corporation, and his position was eliminated. He was generously compensated by the corporation for his job loss and, after calculating the worth of his termination package, John realized that he never needed to work again. In discussing this with his spouse, John decided to use this opportunity to pursue his personal interests including golfing, motorcycling, and recreational boating. However, after one month of living what he referred to as "the good life gone bad," he began to complain about a depressed mood and a sense of hopelessness and stated, "I feel like I have too much time on my hands with nothing to do but watch television, read the newspaper, and worry about all my newly acquired possessions, particularly my boat." John's complaining became so severe that his wife urged him to apply for an accounting job just so he could "get back to normal." It was not long before John was hired by a local accounting firm. Once he had adjusted to his new work schedule, John's emotional problems all but disappeared. He continued, however, to complain that his new job was too time consuming for him to enjoy his family, friends, and leisure pursuits.

Internal continuity is a sense of consistency in one's tendencies and dispositions in old age. Although a given individual may find him- or herself in multiple roles throughout the life span, people are predictable in how they will behave, even in changing external contexts. This predictability was labeled by Atchley as a manifestation of *internal continuity*. Atchley asserts that the basis of internal continuity is the extent to which a person knows who he or she is, or a personal reference point that is within the individual regardless of situations or contexts.

Although internal continuity suggests that a person's past propensities, including his or her values, preferences, attitudes, and world view, are predictive of future behavior, subtle changes that occur as a consequence of incremental learning from personal experiences—both one's mistakes and successes, the observed lives of others, as well as the influence of formal and informal education—can, over time, alter one's basic sense of internal continuity. Interestingly, this kind of gradual change can be almost imperceptible across short intervals of time. Maturation as the force underlying continuity and change, then, is a subtle, but ever-present change-agent within individuals that is actualized as one learns to adapt to the dynamic challenges of living.

External Continuity

The notion of external continuity is different from internal continuity inasmuch as the focus of stability and maturational change is not on internal dispositions or traits, but the external environment. Vivid demonstrations of external continuity are embodied in the kinds of living environments that people create for themselves (Dad's favorite chair). The need to preserve external continuity can be seen in the propensity of some aging parents and grandparents to prefer to spend the holidays in their own home as opposed to traveling to be with family.

As an example of external continuity, it is well known that for many older adults, the loss of one's driver's license can be highly traumatic, even if the negative consequences of driving at advanced age are obvious. However, the loss of one's driver's license may be seen as a restriction of one's ability to manipulate the external environment, particularly as it relates to a person's functional independence. Therefore, to preserve a sense of external continuity an older adult may be adamant about renewing and maintaining an active driver's license even years after he or she has stopped driving.

This propensity to create and maintain stable external structures represents the need for external continuity. Atchley noted, "Continuity of activities, skills, and environments [external continuity] is a logical result of leading to one's strengths to get optimum satisfaction from life" (1989, p. 195). An example of external continuity is highlighted below:

After the death of her spouse, Sally was left with a home that was too large for her to live in alone. However, she was very attached to her home and was stubbornly resistant to consider moving into a smaller apartment or living in the home of one of her children. While her husband Dave was alive, Sally enjoyed inviting her three adult children (and their families) to vacation with them during the various holidays in her home. Sally now feared that if she sold her home these traditions would be lost and this caused her distress. One of her sons suggested that she go through her home and select those items of furniture that meant the most to her and embodied important memories, and he would then rent her an apartment and arrange her chosen furniture so that it would resemble her current home. He noted that there would be predictable differences: this apartment would be smaller, would have no yard, and would be located in a different city. He suggested that she might stay in this apartment for a few weeks at a time to "try it out" and see if she could be comfortable living there. He even suggested that the family arrange a gathering that could occur at this apartment. His plan also involved not selling Sally's home immediately, but letting it remain in Sally's mind, as her primary residence, while this apartment could be a temporary "get away" for her.

Sally reluctantly agreed to this proposal and was further re-assured by the fact that her son agreed that the down payment and security deposit would be a shared cost across Sally's children and that they would also use this apartment when Sally was not living in it. She liked the idea that her house would not be sold and she felt good about decorating the apartment with her existing furniture in a manner she liked and sharing the apartment with her children. She was unwilling to consider it "her" apartment, but indicated that she would try staying in it for a few weeks to compare it to her current living situation. After the new apartment was purchased, the children helped Sally move selected articles of furniture, clothing, and housewares into it. At first, Sally could only stay in the apartment for one or two days after which time she wanted to return home. There were several months when she had some furniture moved back to her home and other furniture moved to the apartment because she was not satisfied with how the apartment looked. The children also helped by providing family photographs and pictures of her grandchildren that they left at the apartment after their stays. Sally began to like the idea of decorating the apartment and she enjoyed looking at the family pictures. Over time, she became accustomed to the apartment and even began to appreciate its advantages. It was, for example, more modern than her home, was easier to up-keep, and was located closer to her children. Within a year, Sally was ready to sell her home and move into her new apartment.

This vignette underscores the need for external continuity in minimizing the distress associated with major change in one's surroundings, particularly when a discontinuity (such as the death of a loved one or the need to move to an assisted living center) threatens to change a very stable living environment. For Sally, her home represented a number of important meanings for her. It was a link to her long-term marriage and a source of positive memories associated with that marriage. The house also represented a gathering place for Sally's children and an important repository of family traditions. Sally did not want to lose these memories, even though the death of her spouse precipitated a change in how the family would view her and her home in the future. Her son understood that giving Sally a chance to gradually experiment with a new living context, knowing that she could always return to her previous home, would lower her threshold of resistance enough to allow Sally to entertain the idea of moving. The goal in this sense was not to pressure Sally to relocate as soon as possible, even though there might be practical and financial advantages to a quick relocation, but to respect Sally's need to remain in her home for as long as she wished. This had the psychological advantage, consistent with continuity theory, of providing her with a way to explore a new living arrangement before committing to a permanent change. In the end, Sally was able to assume control of this move and fully enjoy transitioning to her new living situation.

Together, internal and external continuity represent powerful stabilizing forces of predictability that can be counted on when the challenges and problems of aging arise. However, in order to maximize continuity, limitations on how much change is possible are also important to consider. Thus, in the latter half of the adult life span one could anticipate that both internal and external continuity would be mediating factors in determining how older adults approach tasks that become new in a familiar context (managing the household while caring for a dementing spouse), or how they adapt to changing living situations (moving from independent living to a residential care community), or dealing with personal challenges that are connected to the aging process (age-related disability).

Discontinuity

An important element in continuity theory is the concept of discontinuity that is based on the fact that there are events (internal or external) that occur unexpectedly for the individual. Discontinuities exert their strongest effect when they impact the individual and permanently alter one's sense of stability. Even among those who believe (and act) on the adage that the best laid plans produce the most predictable outcomes, it is almost impossible for an individual to encounter a life situation where a large and unanticipated change will never occur.

When a positive discontinuity occurs, the consequent emotions may include surprise and happiness. A negative discontinuity can produce fear or even depression. Either way, a discontinuity disrupts a person's sense of internal stability. Thus, change (and its subsequent psychological consequences) must be a part of any developmental theory of adulthood. By definition, discontinuity is a break or a separation in either internal or external continuity. Atchley is careful to use a neutral word when describing discontinuity, because, as he notes, a discontinuity not only has the potential for disruption, but it can also be associated with growth or the further maturation of one's worldview and personal capacities. Examples of discontinuities are highlighted below, along with the likely effects on an individual.

The unexpected loss of one's job—(dread) external discontinuity

You let go of a longstanding grudge against a family member—(relief) internal discontinuity

You have an unexpected visit from a friend—(surprise) external discontinuity

You are given a community award that you had not expected, but that involves significant social recognition—(personal satisfaction) external discontinuity

You have a personal/existential crisis in midlife—(anxiety) internal discontinuity

Dealing with discontinuities always requires the investment of personal resources, either for mobilizing information from the past as a way to integrate or construe the change experience in order to reestablish continuity, or the expenditure of effort to come up with novel ideas to facilitate change in one's personal stability. With time, it is the propensity of the older person, given the accumulation of years of living a predictable lifestyle, that even some of the most dramatic and substantial discontinuities will move into the background as the person restabilizes him- or herself so as to regain a sense of balance. However, what may remain when a discontinuity is encountered, even in old age, is a change in one's expectations about the future.

If a person were to have a serious car accident traveling a certain route (an external discontinuity), although the route might not be responsible for the accident, the person might in the future avoid traveling the route because of the expectation (or in this case, the fear) that something unexpected might occur along this route again. The old adage that if you fall off a horse, then get back on immediately, is a strategy that is often proposed to help mitigate a negative schema based on a discontinuity.

At the same time, even in the absence of discontinuity, continuity-mediated change occurs in old age as well. Maturation that was noted earlier is an example of how the qualitative nature of a person's sense of internal and external continuity changes with the passage of time. Atchley asserted that although continuity suggests stability, older adults do have the capacity to change, and in fact, considerable change occurs as one grows older. Positive aging is characterized by stability–change tensions as older adults respond to external pressures or internal processes that require adaptation (Gutmann, 1987).

In sum, Atchley's theory of continuity is based on principles of stability over the life span. Change, or adaptation to change, involves the application of existing psychological resources in new ways to solve problems that present themselves in the future. Problems or issues may be due to internal processes (a sense that one's life is unfulfilled) or external events (the caring for a chronically ill spouse). When unexpected issues arise, a discontinuity occurs. In this case, a person then is compelled to engage in a process of restabilizing his or her sense of consistency in the hope that well-being will return. How this relates to growing old and, in particular, positive aging, is described next.

Continuity Theory and Positive Aging

An unstated but fundamental assumption of continuity theory is that age has a subtle but ever-present influence on one's sense of continuity. For example, everyone must at some point die. Death, then, represents the one ultimate challenge to an individual's continuity, and for this reason people have developed multiple psychological mechanisms to deal with this event. If someone espouses a religious philosophy that affirms life after death, then he or she may feel that living one's life in a positive way may facilitate the continuance of internal continuity, even though the death of one's body represents a profound external discontinuity. Of course, death is only one example of the kinds of events that are a predictable part of aging and that can affect one's sense of continuity, including changes in social status, position in the family, health, or intellectual capability.

Although there is the ever-present desire to postpone (or stop) age-related decline, positive aging involves accepting the reality that age-related deterioration and change is inevitable. A positive aging perspective focuses on the concept that by living into old age it is possible to find a deeper source of meaning and a sense of personal completeness that comes from reflecting over the life that one has lived. This is highlighted in the final stage of Erikson's model (integrity vs. despair) and, with respect to continuity theory, the review of one's life, as it relates to the quality of aging in the present and in the future emerges as one of the most important features of continuity. Malcolm Cowley in his book, *The View from 80*, described this phenomenon eloquently:

> The new octogenarian feels as strong as ever when he is sitting back in a comfortable chair. He ruminates, he dreams, he remembers. He doesn't want to be disturbed by others. It seems to him that old age is only a costume assumed for those others; the true, the essential self is ageless. . . . The body and its surroundings have their messages for him, or only one message: "You are old." (1980, pp. 3–4)

The notion of continuity makes intuitive sense as a description of the nature and course of the aging process. It is a useful heuristic for understanding a dynamic that is involved in maturation as it occurs in old age. However, like Erikson's life stages, it lacks predictive capability; that is, the notion of continuity (and discontinuity) does not lend itself easily to empirical validation and intervention formulation beyond its emphasis on utilizing history (or the past) as a way to enhance coping in the present and future.

Issues in Application

Continuity is, however, a useful guide for counseling because it describes processes that are involved in coping with transitions across the life span. Continuity theory acknowledges that there are specific needs that people have for stability and predictability and these must be balanced against the degree to which a life transition affects one's sense of ongoing stability. Its application to older adults is particularly useful given that the longer one lives, the more disruptive change (or discontinuity) is to one's sense of continuity.

When Steve, at 84, became memory impaired to the point where he was unable to take care of himself at home, his son Dick found a residential care facility that he could move to. Initially Steve was reluctant to move into the facility for fear that he would never come out. He said, "I've lived at home all my life and I want to die there as well." When Steve was admitted to the facility, he was noticeably affected. He lost his appetite, lost interest in engaging in any activity, and was unwilling to leave his room. The care center contacted Dick and suggested that he visit with them about some ideas that might help his father adjust to these new surroundings.

Steve's case is not unlike the issues many adult children face when an elderly parent is unable to live at home and there are no family resources to keep the parent at home or move the parent into the children's own home. The transition to a residential care center can often be traumatic, particularly when a person has had very little experience living outside the home. This was the case with Steve. A continuity intervention might be to establish a link between Steve's home environment and the residential care facility to which he is relocated. Moving Steve back and forth from the facility to home, given his memory impairment, might serve to worsen his condition by creating frequent discontinuities. Therefore, several components of a continuity-sensitive intervention are critical to facilitating Steve's successful transition, including the cooperation of the residential center staff as well as Dick's willingness to engage in efforts to help his father make such a transition.

The steps of a continuity intervention might be as follows:

1. Establish some external linkages between the new residence and Steve's home of origin: When a person relocates he or she may take along meaningful items. Although this seems like an obvious point, it is often overlooked when an elderly person moves into a residential care facility that has its own infrastructure for living. Therefore, the first phase of a continuity intervention would be to introduce some common objects into Steve's living environment to help him feel more at home. This might involve bringing furniture or objects from his home and placing them strategically in his room, including pictures and other objects that would provide significant reminders of home for Steve. If Steve was sufficiently intact intellectually, then it might make sense to find out his preferences about which objects he valued the most.

2. With respect to internal continuity, it would be useful to find out about Steve's likes and dislikes, his favorite activities, his preferred foods, his leisure pursuits, and his hobbies. The goal in this regard is to develop a repertoire of personal likes and dislikes that could be matched with activities at the care center or the introduction of a few specialized activities for Steve to engage in. If Steve enjoyed reading the newspaper on Sundays, he might be provided with a newspaper on a regular basis so that he could keep this routine intact. At a social level, if Steve enjoyed playing bridge at home with his friends and family, this activity might be introduced (or Steve might be encouraged to participate initially with his son Dick in an ongoing bridge game at the care center). This could be a way to build some common linkages between Steve's personal preferences (someone who likes to play games and interact with others) and activities that match his relational style.

3. Another valuable activity to engage in would be to visit with Steve about his likes and dislikes. More often than not, institutions and staff within those institutions tend to forget that residents are real people with real needs who would like to have their needs discussed with them. The burden of care, which can be very great in such contexts, may overshadow the

humanity of the care recipients. In this instance, a continuity intervention should emphasize Steve's participation in as much of the care process and the transition as possible. Steve could be consulted about the temperature of his room, the level of lighting, and the placement of his bed. Even if it were difficult for Steve to provide a fully rational response, the fact that he was being attended to in this way could instill confidence that he was in a setting where his needs and wants were being considered. His sense that he could change his environment to match his personal preferences could enhance his sense of internal continuity.

The strength of using principles of continuity theory in interventions to facilitate physical or emotional adjustments during transitions is apparent. The focus of the intervention is not on Steve as a care burden, but on who Steve is, where he came from, what his preferences are, and how these interact with his care needs. Further, even if Steve was cognitively impaired, the fact that he was being treated in tone and in voice as a person who was worthwhile and able to shape his own environment could ease the challenge of such transitions and mobilize the remaining resources that Steve continues to possess.

SELECTIVITY, OPTIMIZATION, AND COMPENSATION (SOC)

The final theory of adult development and aging, selectivity, optimization, and compensation (SOC), focuses on specific forces that can be isolated to facilitate positive aging (Baltes, 1997). This is, perhaps, the most comprehensive and empirically grounded theory of adult development and aging that exists in the scientific literature specific to gerontology.

Selectivity

Selectivity refers to the process by which individuals become more discriminating in their choice of activities on which to expend time and energy. In general, emphasis is given to endeavors that are more satisfying and highly valued (such as only spending time with family versus spending time with friends, neighbors, and coworkers). This notion of selectivity is embedded in sociopsychological theories such as socioemotional selectivity theory (Carstensen, 1992; Lang & Carstensen, 1994), which posits that older adults reduce their social support network in order to focus their limited (or declining) affiliational resources on only the most important relationships (the nuclear family). This active narrowing of one's social support network would be evidence of selectivity in action through adaptive social disengagement to preserve one's most meaningful relationships.

Optimization

Optimization refers to the processes by which the older adult develops increased functional efficacy via overlearning, practice, and experience in order to continue to perform at a level that was possible when the individual was younger. A considerable body of research has focused on developmental processes of optimization through models of education and learning that are specific to older adults and that can be used to make a person more efficient in performing an intellectual task (Willis, 1985). Intensive memory skill training could be a form of optimization to preserve one's declining memory abilities (Baltes, Dittman-Kohli, & Kliegl, 1986).

Compensation

Compensation is the conscious effort that is employed to mitigate limitations and losses in function associated with the aging process (Bäckman & Dixon, 1992). Culture facilitates the individual's strategic utilization of compensation through advances in technology and science. As an example, it is well known that vision deteriorates in old age. However, eyeglasses are readily available to compensate for age-related deterioration of the natural lens of the eye. There are, of course, numerous other compensatory devices, such as wheelchairs and hearing aids.

Evidence suggests that these three principles of SOC can be used not only to predict the consequences of coping (Bäckman & Dixon, 1992; Freund, Li, & Baltes, 1999; Marsiske, Lang, Baltes, & Baltes, 1995), but can be directly employed in interventions designed to promote positive aging in late life (Baltes & Baltes, 1990; Freund & Baltes, 2002; Schulz, Maddox, & Lawton, 2000).

An important component of SOC is the notion that even in old age people possess a certain degree of internal (or intrapsychic) plasticity, defined as unused intra- and interpersonal resources or reserve capacity, which can be engaged when a person is confronted with a novel situation that involves change in order to adapt (P. B. Baltes, 1993; P. B. Baltes & M. M. Baltes, 1990). P. B. Baltes (1997) noted that the decomposition of the "life span architecture" is not limited to physical function, but includes psychological and intellectual processes as well. Although SOC is somewhat pessimistic in its view of aging, it is indeed a well-established fact, which cannot be ignored in any theory of aging, that the ultimate end of the aging process is death, which is, in the language of SOC, a "normative process of complete decomposition." Thus, the central assumption of SOC is that the balance of developmental gains versus losses inevitably shifts its weight toward the loss side in old and very old age (M. M. Baltes, 1995). The key to SOC, however, is that because each person possesses a degree of untapped stores of internal or dormant reserve capacity, there is variability in how individuals deal with the gain-to-loss shift in the overall aging process, although even this latent capacity diminishes as a function of age and disease, as noted in

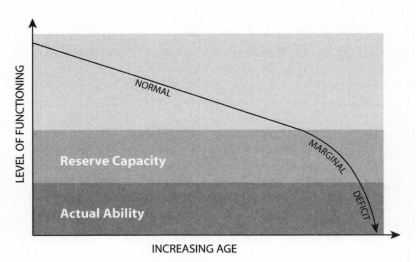

FIGURE 2.2. LATENT CAPACITY DIMINISHES AS A FUNCTION OF AGE.

Figure 2.2. As seen in this figure, functioning is maintained with increasing age even though in old age reserve capacity must be accessed to preserve stable levels of functioning. However, in very old age when the need for reserve capacity increases to maintain homeostasis, and in the presence of finite reserves, functional decline, or changes in observable abilities and behaviors (labeled in this figure as "actual ability"), predictably ensues.

This concept of reserve capacity as a latent (or untapped) resource potential that can mediate age-related decline, has been described by researchers and scholars for decades. In the 1980s, Fries and Crapo (1981) noted that one apparent role of physiological reserve capacity, which occurs in the form of organ redundancy, was a source of latent capability that could be accessed when the human body needed it to maintain stable functioning during conditions of stress or disease. They also noted that this reserve capacity appears to be affected by the aging process inasmuch as it diminishes as one grows older. This has been proffered as one explanation as to why older adults are more susceptible to disability and death due to disease than are younger persons who presumably have more reserves. The notion of reserve capacity has been described for intellectual functioning as well (Stern, 2002); that is, when memory declines are more attenuated in old age in some people, as opposed to others, one explanatory factor could be the existence of greater brain reserve capacity. In those persons who experience smaller decrements in cognitive function as a result of advancing age or disease, it has been postulated that they are accessing reserve capacity to stave off impending decline. The ability of the brain to access neurological structures that are present, but are not functionally engaged, could explain why some people experience less age-related cognitive decline in old age than others. The concept of reserve capacity has implications for understanding individual differences in functionality in older adults and the degree to which older persons can use training or skill enhancement interventions to offset decline. Several researchers have documented that there are interpersonal reserve capacity factors such as social support and socioeconomic status that appear to mediate the negative effects of interpersonal loss in old age (Stroebe, Hansson, Stroebe, & Schut, 2001).

In concert with reserve capacity, SOC theory rests on the conceptual foundation of a two-process model of human functioning: fluid mechanics and crystallized pragmatics (Baltes, 1993). These two processes represent a hydraulic not too dissimilar to the Freudian concept of intrapsychic forces. Fluid mechanics are analogous to a computer's hardware. Baltes has asserted that the hardware of the mind is associated with a person's innate sensory functioning, as well as basic cognitive capabilities such as processing speed, and memory. Crystallized pragmatics, on the other hand, reflect cumulative learning, both formal and informal, of the individual within the context of his or her own culture (Baltes, 1993). Formal education is an example of crystallized pragmatics.

The cognitive mechanics and reserve capacity perspective of SOC are strongly connected to biological and health factors inasmuch as decline is inevitable with advancing age. In some respects, acknowledging such a fact can be a first step to effective coping with late life issues. SOC, in a sense, gives a person permission to experience deterioration and suggests that coping involves making the best of one's experience in old age in the presence of decline. However, an interesting point made by Baltes is that in a few instances, as long as there is sufficient reserve capacity, there may be selective improvements in old age on some abilities. This idea introduces the notion of strategies or techniques that a person can develop in order to optimize her or his functioning. One such strategy could be learning a memory technique (or mnemonic) to reduce the cognitive effort needed to remember a name or a face. This then would have the appearance of improving memory, even in the presence of age-related decline. In several studies of memory performance contrasting old versus young persons, Baltes and his colleagues demonstrated (see Kliegl, Smith, & Baltes et al., 1989; Kliegl, Smith, & Baltes, 1990) that when older adults use strategies, their memory performance improves beyond that of younger untrained persons (with ostensibly more reserve capacity). A memory skills approach to training will be described in detail in Chapter 3. The concept of reserve capacity is presented here as a meaningful component for positive aging, given that a characteristic of positive aging is the ability to access one's reserves, whether they are physiological, cognitive, or social, to address problems and challenges associated with aging. In other words, how one exercises choice and will through tapping latent resources and mobilizing these to cope with challenges, describes positive aging.

Research provides examples of using reserve capacity to promote positive aging. An exercise regime appears to be a mechanism to access physiological reserve capacity that then mediates bone loss in older women with osteoporosis (Bravo, Gauthier, Roy, and Payette, 1996). Older adults who have greater socioeconomic status or those who have cultivated a rich social support network, appear to be able to deal better with interpersonal losses than are those who are unable to access these sources of interpersonal reserve capacity (Gallo, Bogart, Vranceanu, Matthews, 2005). Some research suggests that years of formal schooling provide cognitive reserves to attenuate the progressive nature of Alzheimer's disease (Springer, McIntosh, Winocur, Grady, 2005).

This three-component mechanism of selectivity, optimization, and compensation contributes to the high degree of individual variability in old age, and Baltes provides substantial evidence that this is the case with respect to psychological functioning. What follows is a brief description of how each of these components of SOC promotes positive aging (Baltes, Staudinger, & Lindenberger, 1999).

SOC and Positive Aging

Positive aging is related to how well the individual applies the three mechanisms of selectivity, optimization, and compensation to ameliorate loss. From Baltes's perspective, a distinction can be made between normal and successful aging depending on how effectively a person applies these mechanisms. In successful aging, Baltes has shown that it is even possible to temporarily suspend or even reverse age-related losses through high levels of training and practice that accesses substantial reserve capacity, and can be sustained as long as reserve capacity remains (Baltes & Baltes, 1990).

Positive aging is descriptive of the phenomenon of the effective employment of strategies to maximize coping and adaptation. However, positive aging also encompasses a psychological component; that is, a perception that through the engagement of SOC a person builds confidence that it is still possible to maintain functioning even in the presence of age-related loss. This change in mindset about the nature of control over age-related decline is essential as a motivating force for engaging in and refining the SOC processes.

The application of SOC, whether to maintain a skill, preserve one's social network, sustain oneself in the presence of a chronic age-related illness, or recover from a dramatic psychological trauma, represents the essential mechanisms for preserving a sense of positive aging into old and very old age.

Issues in Application

Because SOC describes specific mechanisms for adapting to the environment, it is the most testable of the three theories presented in this chapter. For this reason, it can be readily employed as a conceptual framework for addressing a wide variety of problems and issues in old age and then testing, empirically, whether such strategies are effective in changing targeted outcomes (Baltes, Baltes, Freund & Lang, 1999). With respect to what makes SOC work, the more effective an individual is at employing the processes of selectivity, optimization, and compensation to facilitate adaptation, the better a person will deal with the challenges and issues of growing old.

To test this assumption, Cignac, Cott, and Badley (2002) examined whether SOC behaviors could facilitate adaptation to osteoarthritis in 248 older community-dwelling adults with this diagnosis. They defined selection as strategic restriction of activities (withdrawing from field trips that involved extended walking). Optimization was defined as enhancing access to one's reserve capacity by engaging in a program of regular physical exercise to remain fit and minimize pain. Compensation was defined as the propensity to discover alternative means to sustain mobility when impairment was present (using an assistive device such as a walking aid).

The study involved extensive interviews of the participants with respect to how well they employed these SOC principles across 24 activities that would be influenced by their disease (e.g., getting out of bed, preparing meals). These researchers found that almost every older participant engaged in at least one SOC behavior. Compensation was the most frequently reported strategy; however, the ability to engage in one or more SOC behaviors was positively associated with better coping and enhanced quality of life. The more people engaged in SOC behaviors the better they coped with their chronic disease and the more well-being they experienced. In a sense, those who were better at employing SOC experienced a higher level of positive aging even though they were challenged with a progressive chronic deteriorative disease.

CONCLUDING COMMENTS

This chapter has provided an overview of three prominent theories of aging and adult development: Erikson's life stages of psychosocial development, continuity theory, and Baltes et al.'s theory of selection, optimization, and compensation (SOC). These models of aging provide a framework descriptive of positive aging. In regard to developmental theories, positive aging is a psychological state that emphasizes meaning, adaptation, and skill development that is tailored to the qualitative experience of growing old. Enhanced well-being in old age depends on how well a person can find meaning in his or her own aging experience, adapt to changes as these emerge in late life, and develop a repertoire of skills that can be used to mitigate age-related deterioration.

Chapter 3

AGE-RELATED DECLINE
AND ITS EFFECTS

MOST PEOPLE LIVING BEYOND 50 years of age will experience intra- and interpersonal change associated with the aging process. Understanding and helping clients deal with age-related change requires examining the phenomenon not only from the point of view of loss as it is emphasized in SOC (from Chapter 2), but also from the role that age-related change plays in facilitating positive qualities in old age. For some people, years of living and experience can broaden their, perspectives about life and its meaning. Wisdom (referred to by Erikson, see Chapter 2) is ascribed to those persons who are exceptionally good at learning life's lessons and then applying that learning to issues in everyday living. Wisdom is a latent intellectual skill in old age that emerges from a positive aging lifestyle. Unlike cognitive decline, wisdom-related intelligence is acquired by a selective subset of older persons through the process of aging.

TRAJECTORIES OF AGE-RELATED DECLINE

Several groups were introduced in Chapter 1; namely, successful, normal, and diseased agers. An essential aspect of understanding these categories of aging requires juxtaposing them to their characteristic trajectories of decline. Researchers suggest that although all people will experience age-related deficits in later life, there are qualitatively discrete groups of older persons with specific patterns of decline.

- Optimal/Successful Aging: Those who don't decline appreciably (or only minimally) with the passage of time (Hill, Wahlin, et al., 1995; Newman et al., 2003; Seeman et al., 1994).
- Normal Aging: Those whose decline is typical for an individual within a given cultural group (Rowe & Kahn, 1987; Sehl & Yages, 2001).
- Impaired or Deficit Aging: Progressive decline due to physiological impairment that has not reached the diagnostic threshold for disease but operates on the individual by reducing the capacity of the person to function optimally. (Petersen et al., 1999).
- Diseased Aging: Decline resulting in functional impairment due to cardiovascular disease, Alzheimer's, or cancer that produces substantial deficits which interact with the aging process itself (e.g., accelerated aging; Mitnitski, Graham, Mogliner, & Rockwood, 1999).

As can be seen in Figure 3.1 decline can be depicted with respect to the three general markers of longevity described in Chapter 1, average life expectancy (ALE), optimum life potential (OLP), and maximum life span (MLS). However, for each trajectory of decline the age range in which death will most likely occur differs.

Successful aging involves minimal decline that only becomes noticeable after a person exceeds his or her OLP. However, when a person advances (in years) beyond her or his OLP, deterioration begins, and decline becomes more precipitous because the person has moved closer to his or her maximum life span limit. The confidence interval within which death occurs in successful aging is narrow due to the fact that death occurs when a person approaches (or reaches) his or her biological determined age limit.

Normal aging, on the other hand, initially follows a more gradual negative trajectory, although even in normal aging, once OLP is reached, decline accelerates. A distinguishing characteristic of normal aging is the greater variability of trajectories of decline among individuals within this group, hence the much larger

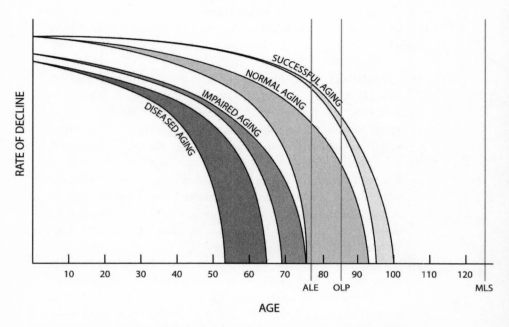

FIGURE 3.1. TRAJECTORY OF DECLINE WITH RESPECT TO ALE, OLP, AND MLS.

  ALE (Average Life Expectancy = 77 Years)
  OLP (Optimum Life Potential = 85 Years)
  MLS (Maximum Life Span = 125 Years)

confidence interval noted in Figure 3.1 for this group. In impaired and diseased aging, decline begins earlier and is more marked than in normal or successful aging. This early decline in impaired aging occurs due to the emergence of pathological conditions or precursory disease symptoms such as fatigue, reduced capacity for activity or intellectual functioning, and diminishment in reserve capacity (Fries & Crapo, 1981). When disease becomes observable or when impairment exceeds the threshold for a disease diagnosis, there is an increase in the slope of decline. This can be seen in Figure 3.1 by contrasting the trajectories of decline for the impaired versus the diseased age trajectory groupings.

Disease not only restricts absolute longevity, meaning the overall percentage of individuals living into very old age is much lower than in the nondiseased groups, but it also influences the variability of individual aging. Diseased aging not only results in reduced longevity outcomes, but once the disease becomes a prominent force that controls decline, the person's deterioration over time becomes more predictable and progressive based on the disease process itself or its interaction with advancing age rather than on aging per se. (Mitnitski et al., 1999).

Regardless of one's trajectory of age-related decline, deficits in cognitive functioning are inevitable in old age and it is one of the most pervasive and ubiquitous concerns that older adults experience as they age (Small, 2001). Cognitive function in this sense involves a number of abilities, including short- and long-term memory, perceptual motor speed, reasoning, and language. For some persons, cognitive decline in old age may be relatively small while for others it may have a profound impact on whether a person can maintain independent functioning in old age. Because age-related cognitive decline is progressive in nature, it is likely that cognitive deficits that impair day-to-day functioning will occur and worsen as a person ages.

AGE-RELATED COGNITIVE DECLINE

It is well established in the gerontological literature that old age involves observable deficits in cognitive function. In the late 1950s, Kral introduced the term *benign senescent forgetfulness* to describe the array of memory complaints that he observed among his older patients who were otherwise free of brain disease (Kral, 1958). Kral noted in these early writings that not only were memory problems more prevalent in old age, but that as any given individual ages, memory problems tend to get worse, and that this is the case even when disease is not present. Since Kral, there has been substantial epidemiological and clinical research that has examined the nature and scope of age-related memory decline (Kausler, 1994). Several general reviews have been published in the scientific literature that summarize decades of research on this topic (Craik, Anderson, Kerr, & Li, 1995; Kausler, 1994; Luszcz & Bryan, 1999; Salthouse, 1991; Schaie, 1995). This research suggests that as people age, not only do memory processes deteriorate, and the likelihood increases that memory deficits will impact everyday functioning, but individual characteristics of a person, such as gender, number of years of formal schooling, and verbal ability, interact with this process (Park, 1992; R. L. West, Crook, & Barron, 1992; Hill, Wahlin, Winblad, & Bäckman, 1995).

One of the first terms to emerge from the scientific literature that gave credence to memory deficits in late life that were not specific to a disease state, was the term *age-associated memory impairment* (AAMI; Crook et al., 1986). AAMI is now a formal label in the *Diagnostic and Statistical Manual of Mental Disorders* (American Psychiatric Association, 1994) and is described as follows:

> [A]n objectively identified decline in cognitive functioning consequent to the aging process that is within normal limits given the person's age. Individuals with this condition may report problems remembering names or appointments. . . . This category should be considered only after it has been determined that the cognitive impairment is not attributable to a specific mental disorder or neurological condition. (p. 684)

The diagnostic criteria for AAMI are: 50 years of age or older; a gradual onset of memory complaints; memory test performance at least one standard deviation below younger people; good intellectual functioning; no diagnosis of dementia; no history of neurological or cerebrovascular disorders. The symptoms of AAMI include a specific pattern of complaints about memory inefficiency in everyday living. Typical everyday tasks such as household management, shopping, conducting business in one's community, interacting with acquaintances, friends, and family, driving a car, or planning for the future, all require some memory capacity, and become more difficult in the presence of AAMI. The feature of AAMI that distinguishes it from disease is the fact that cognitive decline is not as progressive as it is in diseased aging (Crook et al., 1986).

A related and more diagnostically sensitive term, *minimal cognitive impairment* (MCI; Davis & Rockwood, 2004), has replaced AAMI with a definition that includes the possibility that diminished memory function may also foretell a disease process such as Alzheimer's disease or other forms of dementia. Annual prevalence estimates for MCI range from 17 to 34% among adults over 60 years (Peterson, 2000). A person who is diagnosed with MCI may either be experiencing normative, benign changes in memory functioning due to aging or might be experiencing a disease that is moving from the sub-clinical to a clinical or observable (and diagnosable) threshold. It has been estimated that as many as one third of those with MCI will eventually be diagnosed with dementia (Petersen et al., 1999; Wilson, Beckett, Bennett, Albert, & Evans, 1999).

Signs of MCI suggestive of benign senile forgetfulness or normative cognitive decline are: forgetting an unfamiliar phone number after only a few rehearsals of the number; forgetting names of acquaintances; forgetting a few items on a shopping list; misplacing keys occasionally; misplacing a wallet or handbag; wondering whether the door was locked after leaving home.

Early signs of MCI suggestive of disease or impaired aging include forgetting important appointments even with reminders; forgetting to turn off the stove multiple times; getting lost in familiar places such as one's home or neighborhood; getting lost while driving a familiar route such as to the local grocery store; repeating questions over and over, even when the answers to these questions are provided several times in succession; difficulty understanding words; difficulty finding the right words when speaking (Peterson, Stevens, Gangull, Tangalos, Cummings, & DeKosky, 2001).

Distinguishing normal age-related memory deficits from disease processes is a difficult and perplexing problem for several reasons. First, the precise mechanism that causes normative age-related decline is not well understood; however, there is some research which suggests that with advancing age certain predictable physiological changes occur in the brain including size shrinkage and atrophy of brain structures (Kemper, 1994). In addition to these structural changes, functional aspects of the brain deteriorate as well, including slowed metabolism and decreases in existing neurotransmitter levels critical to neuronal communication including dopamine, acetylcholine, and serotonin (Clegg et al., 2001). Interestingly, these changes in brain function and structure have been found to be only loosely associated with brain–behavior relationships.

Second, like the trajectories of decline, individual variability in cognitive functioning in older persons who are aging normally is substantial. For this reason, it is difficult to predict the severity and rate of cognitive decline in any given person, and even harder to determine whether a pattern of decline is due to disease or is simply a variant of normal aging. If, however, change in cognitive performance on a standardized measure of memory or intellectual function moves from the normal into the pathological range, this is evidence that a disease process is present. Practitioners who are working with adults who are concerned about their memory or other deficiencies in cognitive functioning may want to consider obtaining measures of cognitive function across multiple measurement intervals.

Whether cognitive deficits are due to disease or a consequence of normal aging, the qualitative nature of memory and related cognitive problems in older persons is important for the practitioner to understand, given that this is a central issue of concern for many older adults. In a study conducted by Karen Bolla and colleagues at Johns Hopkins University (Bolla, Lindgren, Bonaccorsy, & Bleecker, 1991), 199 adults ranging in age between 39 and 89 years were asked to respond to questions about the impact that memory problems were having on their lives. In addition, these researchers were interested in how closely these complaints were linked to objective tests of memory performance. The findings from this study documented, among other things, that across 13 everyday tasks, four of these, including remembering names and faces, forgetting where items were placed, remembering telephone numbers, and finding the right word to describe objects, were endorsed as problems by more than 50% of the participants. Remembering names and faces was viewed as especially difficult for over 80% of the participants who indicated that this was a problem that affected the quality of their lives. The percentage of individuals from this study endorsing these memory problems is depicted in Figure 3.2, along with a group of 72 older volunteers (60 years and older) at the University of Utah in Salt Lake City, Utah, who were asked the same questions as those in the Bolla study. The Utah participants indicated concerns similar to the Johns Hopkin's University Study participants. The scientific literature is unambiguous in documenting that persons who are 50 years and older will complain about memory problems (Bolla et al., 1991; Verhaeghen, Geraerts, & Marcoen, 2000).

What is surprising about Bolla's findings, however, is that she reported the memory problems in her participants were not as related to objective memory performance as they were to their mood state. In other words, her participants' scores on a self-report depression survey were more closely tied to their memory complaints than they were to their actual performance on a battery of memory and other cognitive

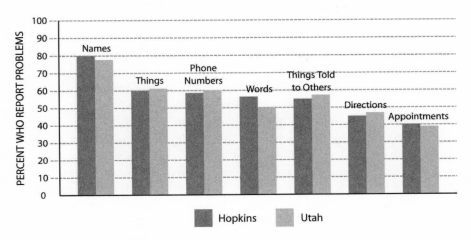

FIGURE 3.2. PERCENTAGE OF INDIVIDUALS ENDORSING MEMORY PROBLEMS. (ADAPTED FROM BOLLA ET AL., 1991. UTAH DATA IS UNPUBLISHED.)

ability tests. This finding is consistent with the general theme in the scientific literature which suggests that the nature of cognitive decline in old age is as associated with one's psychological state as it is to actual functional memory ability (Blazer, Hays, Fillenbaum, & Gold, 1997; Christensen, 1991; Verhaeghen et al., 2000).

LATE-LIFE MEMORY DECLINE

A first step in articulating a positive aging strategy that evaluates age-related memory decline is to determine whether a given set of symptoms or complaints is due either to AAMI (or MCI without disease features) or to an emerging disease state such as Alzheimer's disease or some other form of dementia (Barnes, 1998). If decline is being driven by disease, the earlier that this can be determined the greater the chance that treatments for the disease will be effective. Therefore, in disease-related memory decline, early detection of the disease is of central importance. Strategies for early detection of disease described in the clinical and scientific literature have ranged from specialized paper-and-pencil screening instruments that assess objective memory performance (Mattis, 1988; Mundt, Freed, & Greist, 2000) to physiological indicators of the disease including biomarkers obtained from blood tests, urine samples, and in some cases, cerebrospinal fluid (Csernansky, Miller, McKeel, & Morris, 2002). It is speculated that these biomarkers may be able to identify the presence of a disease before full-blown disease symptoms emerge (Boller & Katzman, 1989). Unfortunately, biomarkers reliable enough to achieve this objective have not been found, although research continues with great intensity in this area.

What may be most helpful to the practitioner whose role it is to alert a client to the likelihood that memory problems may be due to an emergent disease state (and not just a consequence of normal aging) are self-report or observational measures that can be easily administered and that flag aspects of memory impairment that might be suspicious of disease. This will then be the basis for referring a client to receive more definitive diagnostic medical testing. Although detecting disease from observable behavior is a challenging task, several instruments exist to achieve this objective. The Symptoms of Dementia Screener (SDS; Mundt et al., 2000) is an assessment that identifies behavioral deficits characteristic of dementia through a series of strategic and graded questions about everyday activities that involve cognitive abilities. They are paraphrased below. This instrument is designed to be completed by a caregiver and/or someone who interacts on a day-to-day basis with the client:

- Repeats the same question over and over.
- Is forgetful and has trouble with short-term memory.
- Forgets appointments, family occasions, or holidays.
- Has trouble doing calculations, managing finances, or balancing the checkbook.
- Has lost interest in usual activities such as hobbies, reading, church, and social activities.
- Has started needing help eating, dressing, bathing, or using the bathroom.
- Has become irritable, agitated, or suspicious or started seeing, hearing, or believing things that are not real.
- There is concern about this person's driving, including getting lost or driving unsafely.
- Has trouble finding the words to express him- or herself, including difficulty finishing sentences or naming people or things.

Responses to each question follow a yes or no format. Scoring instructions for this instrument recommend that a threshold sum score (e.g., five yes points or greater) would indicate that a disease process might be present. However, it may be advisable for a practitioner to refer a client for additional diagnostic testing if the client's caregiver endorses enough of these items to exceed a threshold for the client. The SDS is copyrighted, and can be obtained by consulting the source article for this instrument (Mundt et al., 2000).

Strategies for Disease-Related Memory Decline

Once a disease is present, there are only a limited number of strategies for mediating the progression of memory deficits due to disease-related aging. Two of them are: (1) drug therapy and (2) a behavioral strategy called spaced retrieval.

Drug therapy is, by far, the most popular treatment for memory deficits due to dementia. One form of drug treatment that has shown some promise for remediating memory deficits in diseased aging relies on pharmacological agents that work to sustain levels of acetylcholine, a neurotransmitter that is present between neuronal synapses in the brain, and has been found to be associated with memory functioning. Persons with dementia show substantial deficits in acetylcholine and drugs known as acetylcholine inhibitors slow the loss of this neurotransmitter in the diseased brain. Examples of this class of drugs are: donepezil/*Aricept* (Rogers & Friedhoff, 1998); rivastigmine/*Exelon* (Farlow, Anand, Messina, Hartman, & Veach, 2000); and galantamine/*Reminy* (Tariot et al., 2000). Pharmacological treatment has been associated with some success in remediating memory deficits in dementia, although there is also literature indicating that these drugs may not be as effective as originally thought (Clegg et al., 2001). In this regard, the search for more effective drugs continues. Roy Jones (2000) provides an excellent overview and guide to drug treatment for memory deficits in dementia.

Spaced retrieval, pioneered by Cameron Camp (Camp & Stevens, 1990) is an innovative psychological technique that uses progressively spaced repetitions of to-be-remembered information to help an older person who is memory impaired remember important information. In spaced retrieval, the spacing or repetition of information is the key.

Specifically, the retrieval interval is systematically increased until a person is able to recall, from memory, target information for longer time intervals. A patient with Alzheimer's disease may be prompted to remember the name of a family member by repeating the family member's name and recalling the name at intervals that are, at first, very short (e.g., the name is repeated and recalled every 10 seconds), and then are slowly lengthened until the person can repeat the newly learned name after a space of a few minutes to a few hours, to several days. This strategy is labor intensive and is effective for specific information such as remembering the name of a family member or a specific phone number. However, such a strategy does not treat the underlying disease state so, inevitably, as the disease progresses the recall of information that is learned through spaced-retrieval techniques will be lost.

In addition to spaced retrieval, some studies have suggested that memory aids or mnemonics might be effective for improving selected cognitive deficits in demented persons (Hill, Evancovich, Sheikh, & Yesavage, 1987). However, the research literature on the use of mnemonics with older demented adults is equivocal with respect to showing meaningful improvements in memory functioning in demented persons. (Bäckman, Josephsson, Herlitz, Stigsdotter, Uiitanen, 1991).

In diseased aging, because memory functioning is primarily influenced by the course and severity of the disease process and not the rate of aging, remedial memory strategies will ultimately break down as the disease severity increases. This is not the case for normal aging, however, where strategy training and memory techniques can be quite helpful in addressing the effects of memory problems on everyday functioning.

Strategies for Addressing Age-related Memory Decline

If age-related decline in memory functioning is due to normal aging and not a disease process, evaluating the nature of the specific problem with the goal of developing the most effective strategy for treatment would represent the second step in a positive aging approach. In this regard, SOC fits nicely within this scheme because most intervention approaches that have been developed to help older persons deal with age-related memory decline have involved some aspect of SOC.

In terms of selectivity, a positive aging approach to mitigate memory problems in old age is to strategically limit or restrict the amount of new information that one needs to remember in order to accomplish a given task. It may not be necessary, for example, to commit multiple telephone numbers of acquaintances and family members to memory. Instead, one might record phone numbers in an address book or in a personal digital assistant (PDA). In old age, as routines become more circumscribed it makes sense to let old memories fade in order to preserve resources for that smaller subset of essential information needed in everyday functioning. In Bolla's study (Bolla et al., 1991), she asked her participants about reminder techniques they used and how frequently they used them to help recall information. Written documentation was the most frequently used method and these included: (1) keeping an appointment book— 69%; (2) making a grocery list—62%; and (3) making lists of places to go when on an errand—59%. List making and developing a routine that involves thinking about a task before one begins to act may be difficult at first. However, making written lists of what one needs to purchase at the grocery store may have added benefits, such as encouraging the shopper to plan ahead for what he or she needs to purchase. Further, if one has a list while grocery shopping the chances of engaging in impulse buying or spending time inefficiently searching for items will be reduced. The time and effort needed to create a list can make one a more selective and efficient shopper.

To apply the second SOC mechanism, optimization, to address memory problems encountered in old age, a person might work to enhance his or her psychological or intellectual functioning in order to maximize memory capability. There is a growing research literature suggesting that a lifestyle which includes active engagement in intellectual activity preserves memory function in old age (Arbuckle, Gold, Andres, Schwartzman, & Chaikelson, 1992; Hill, Wahlin et al., 1995). In a large-scale longitudinal study of 250 older adults from the Victoria Longitudinal Study in British Columbia, Canada, participants were assessed over a 6- and 18-month time period on a battery of memory and related cognitive ability tasks (Hultsch et al., 1999). They were also queried, in depth, about 70 different kinds of everyday activities that they engaged in. This study found evidence supporting the idea that engaging in mentally stimulating activities including reading, crossword puzzles, and board games that challenge verbal or memory ability, aided in preserving memory and intellectual functioning in the presence of age-related decline. These were, for the most part, very healthy older adults who were not only highly educated but relatively affluent and living or vacationing in Victoria, British Columbia, so there are a number of variables, such as the excellent physical health of these participants and their access to medical care, that could have explained these findings; however, the hypothesis that mental activity buffers age-related cognitive decline has been found in numerous studies from other groups of older adults, so these findings are generally supportive of this literature and illustrative of the idea that optimizing one's intellectual skill through active engagement in mental activities may buffer the negative effects of aging on memory function.

Research has also suggested that a lifestyle involving active intellectual pursuits may even be protective of Alzheimer's disease. In one study that was reported in the *New England Journal of Medicine* (Verghese et al., 2003), researchers followed 469 older persons across a 21-year period with ongoing assessments of their mental functioning and their lifestyle and leisure pursuits. Intellectual leisure tasks included reading, doing puzzles, playing mental manipulation games, and mentally challenging activities. When these activities were quantified with respect to time spent engaging in them, those who represented the top third of participants had a 63% lower risk of dementia in comparison to those who represented the bottom third on this measure. They also postulated that engaging in a mentally stimulating activity once per day every week reduced the risk of dementia by 7%. These findings underscore the importance of optimization of one's intellectual resources as a positive aging strategy to remediate age-related memory decline.

Optimization in the form of maintaining one's intellectual skills through a lifestyle of cognitive engagement may be important to recommend as a strategy to sustain not only one's mental abilities into old age, but to provide a buffer against age-related cognitive diseases such as dementia. It is important to note that in optimization, the goal is to enhance one's overall capability to function rather than teaching a focused skill to remediate a specific problem. The latter approach represents compensation, which is perhaps the most substantial area for memory remediation in older persons who are experiencing age-associated memory impairment (or MCI without disease features present). Learning a remedial memory skill through training fits within the compensation dimension of SOC because it involves learning and applying compensatory memory techniques designed to offset memory deficits in old age. Compensation refers to the application of interventions designed to teach skills that can offset deficits by specifically targeting the deficit. Strategy training, assistive technology, or the creation of supportive conditions that can compensate for areas where functioning has been lost, are all descriptive of the SOC mechanism of compensation.

MEMORY TRAINING: SKILL-BASED COMPENSATION FOR MEMORY DECLINE

Memory training as a skill-based compensation strategy involves learning a specific technique (called a mnemonic) that is designed to enhance remembering through either improving the organization of the information to be recalled (organizational mnemonics) or mentally linking information to be recalled to more familiar mental images that are stored in the learner's permanent (or long-term) memory. In the latter case, recalling a familiar image becomes the cue for retrieving the newly learned information from memory.

Research has documented that certain kinds of memory training techniques can directly compensate for memory deficits in older persons. A mnemonic called the Method of Loci (Kliegl, Smith, & Baltes, 1989, 1990), when implemented by older adults, has been found to produce substantial gains in memory performance, especially if the training was at a sufficient level to help one to become a proficient user of this technique. The Method of Loci involves the creation of discrete mental images that link information that a person desires to remember (the name of an acquaintance) with a location or a place that is familiar to the learner. The to-be-learned name would be mentally linked to the familiar location, which would act as a cue for the name. To remember the name, a person would

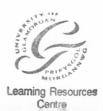

mentally imagine the location, and once it was recalled, the to-be-remembered information (in this case the person's name) would be retrieved using the familiar location as a cue. For example, to memorize items that one needs to pick up at a hardware store (nails, shovel, glue, etc.), a person would first develop a set of loci or familiar locations in one's house; namely the front door, the light in the hallway, the bed in the bedroom, the television set in the bedroom, and so on. It is then that one would mentally place each to-be-remembered object in a specific location (for example, the nails sticking into the door or glue stuck to the hall light). The object is to train oneself to mentally travel to each landmark and then visualize the to-be-remembered object.

Although substantial research has accumulated in support of the efficacy of the Method of Loci as a memory aid (Kliegl et al., 1989, 1990), its practical value for dealing with everyday memory problems is somewhat limited. It could be used to help a person commit a grocery shopping list to memory, or a list of items that one might need to obtain during an errand. It is significant that research using the Method of Loci with older persons has shown that mnemonics can be learned by the elderly who can use them to compensate for memory deficits and, in a limited set of circumstances, even improve memory functioning by accessing mental reserve capacity (Baltes, Dittman-Kohli & Kliegl, 1986; Kliegl, Smith & Baltes, 1989).

How to Remember a PIN

It is becoming increasingly difficult to access services without using PINs and other numeric passwords for use with ATMs or the Internet. The degree to which older adults use such services and maintain security, may depend on their ability to retrieve a specific number combination at the point of service (e.g., standing in front of an ATM). Because remembering numbers is difficult at any age, the inability to recall a PIN may prevent older persons from making optimal use of such services.

Although a PIN could be written down, to do so poses a security risk. This type of issue is an excellent context for employing a mnemonic as a SOC compensation strategy. One specific technique for recalling a number sequence is called the "number-consonant-mnemonic." It has been used in several empirical investigations to enhance memorizing number strings in both younger (Higbee, 1988) and older (Hill, Campbell, Foxley, & Lindsay, 1997) persons. There are four steps to this mnemonic:

The first step involves memorization of digit-to-letter pairs; namely, 1 = l, 2 = n, 3 = m, 4 = r, 5 = f or v, 6 = b or d, 7 = k or hard c, 8 = t, 9 = p or g, 0 = s or z or soft c. It is essential that these digit-letter pairs are completely learned. This can be done by linking the letter and the number to a common physical characteristic or a sound (i.e., 2 = n because n has 2 down strokes; 4 ends with the sound *r*).

The second step involves transcribing the to-be-remembered numerical sequence (or the digits) to their corresponding consonants and then combining the letters with placeholder vowels to form a word or series of words that can then be memorized. The number sequence 2410, for example, would be transcribed to the four letters *NRLS*. By interspersing vowels or other silent consonants among these vocalized consonants, a meaningful word or series of words can be created (NeaR LoSs).

The third step involves committing the created word or word series to memory. This can be done by selecting words that are connected to the number sequence in some meaningful way. For example, to remember the ATM PIN 0532 the phrase *SaVe MoNey* might be created.

These steps are a brief description of how to apply the mnemonic technique to remember number sequences. A fuller description of this strategy and how it is used can be found in several self-help memory training books (Higbee, 1989; West, 1985). This mnemonic is presented here, primarily as an example of a memory strategy SOC technique that can be learned to help in daily living situations that require numeric recall.

The Method of Loci and the Number-Consonant-Mnemonic are both specific techniques for learning and remembering certain kinds of materials. In this sense, they are excellent examples of compensatory strategies. There are a large number of mnemonics that can be tailored to specific information including the name-face mnemonic for remembering a person's name and face, and the method of loci mnemonics described earlier for remembering lists and objects that one might need to buy or collect. It is useful for the practitioner who works with older adults to be familiar with strategies such as these that can help an older client with certain kinds of problems or issues due to late-life memory loss.

WISDOM AS A POSITIVE OUTCOME OF AGE-RELATED CHANGE

A positive outcome of age-related change for some older persons is the acquiring of wisdom. Recall from Chapter 2 that Erikson described wisdom as a consequence of resolving the life-stage development of "integrity vs. despair." Erikson believed that wisdom is a kind of maturity that helps a person to reconcile his or her own reality with what the person desires to accomplish in the remaining years of living. In this sense, wisdom is the mature implementation of selectivity (from SOC) as a way to get the most out of one's remaining years of living. A wisdom perspective includes helping others as well as promoting a greater understanding for oneself about the meaning and purpose of life. Wisdom is only obtainable through life experience, and for this reason the longer one lives, the more wisdom may be developed. People who are wise can often be found as the central figures in social or family groups, not necessarily because a wise person is one who makes the rules or gives orders, but because one of the elements of wisdom is the ability to teach or help others find sources of well-being and satisfaction in life (Staudinger, Smith & Baltes, 1992).

Wisdom can be learned even when one's memory and other cognitive skills are in decline. So, it is fitting to discuss wisdom as representing one of the consequences of effectively coping with cognitive loss in old age. Wisdom could be construed as the advanced application of SOC strategies to tap reserve capacity and address cognitive deficits as well as build an expert skill set in how to live life.

In the scientific literature, wisdom has been studied not only as a developmental construct that embodies features of positive aging, but also as an outcome of everyday learning that produces a specialized form of intelligence that gets refined through the process of making decisions, experiencing the outcome of those decisions, and learning from one's mistakes and successes over the course of a lifetime (Sternberg, 1990). Baltes (1993) defines wisdom as "an expert knowledge system in the fundamental pragmatics of life permitting excellent judgment and advice involving important and uncertain matters of life" (p. 586). The idea that wisdom is acquired through knowledge suggests that it is a consequence of a learning-oriented process of living. However, it is a kind of learning that requires a deeper understanding of the features of the world including its "unknowns" and "uncertainties." For example, tragedies and difficulties in living do not always conform to one's limited expectations, and those people who are able to develop a relativistic approach to failure and disappointment, including being able to learn from every kind of experience, are the more likely candidates for developing wisdom.

Some researchers have suggested that if wisdom is a skill, it should be possible to teach people to be wise. Researchers and scholars who have studied wisdom have highlighted five skills that define wisdom, including the capability to: (1) purposefully examine one's own life to actualize self-improvement; (2) resolve dilemmas and make decisions that promote life satisfaction; (3) advise others in such a way as to promote their well-being; (4) engage in managing and guiding individuals and groups within a social or community system without diminishing individual choice and freedom; and (5) genuinely question the meaning of life with the idea that different people find happiness through multiple sources of meaning (Kramer, 1990).

As these five capabilities attest, wisdom may manifest itself in some people as a kind of learning that occurs as a product of the interplay of maturational forces and specific life events. As a consequence, a wise person becomes proficient in cultivating optimism through good decision making, and in espousing an orientation that is "other" focused or that is altruistic in terms of how one views the needs of others. In support of these characteristics, Holliday and Chandler (1986) asked approximately 500 persons of all ages to identify features of wisdom in individuals whom they considered wise. This research produced some common themes or descriptors of a wise person including older age, exceptional understanding, superior judgment, general competence in decision making, excellent communication skills, and social ease.

Although aging (or simply growing old) does not necessarily mean that a person will become wise, it is clear that a critical feature of wisdom is that it is a life span characteristic that emerges from the ability to learn from one's experiences whether these are good or bad. From the point of view of SOC, wisdom could be characterized as a way of optimizing one's aging in order to offset age-related decline by cultivating an approach to living that involves engaged and proactive adaptation. The better a person meets the challenges of age-related decline the more likely that person could be characterized as wise.

Like Holiday and Chandler, Baltes and colleagues also conducted a series of studies with older people who were nominated as wise by influential persons in the area of Berlin, Germany (Baltes & Staudinger, 2000; Baltes, Staudinger, Maercker, & Smith, 1995). These persons were then invited to participate in a series of experiments to elucidate the component skills of wisdom. Specifically, they were asked to respond to two vignettes designed to tap wisdom-related decision-making skills; namely, a life planning issue (a woman attempting to reconcile conflict between her desire to begin a late-life career and her family responsibilities) and an existential life crisis (the expressed threat of suicide by a friend despondent over the lack of meaning in life). The responses of these wise persons were contrasted to two control groups of older and younger persons respectively who were intelligent (as defined by their performance on a test of intelligence and verbal skill), but were not considered (through nomination by persons within the Berlin community) as wise. The wisdom group outperformed the younger and older non-wisdom controls by coming up with more optimal solutions to the vignette dilemmas. Baltes concluded that: (1) wisdom does not appear to deteriorate with age, and in fact, aging may be a precondition of wisdom; (2) specific life-span learning conditions facilitate wisdom. Among these were: superior knowledge about what really matters in everyday living; knowledge of "how" to solve life problems along with the ability to teach problem-solving strategies to others; an appreciation of the relative nature of one's goals and aspirations and the need to modify personal goals from time to time; an awareness that although there is uncertainty in life it is possible to find optimal solutions to problems of living; and an awareness of one's own value system and how it is similar and different to the values of others.

Given the view of wisdom as a life span skill, it may be that professionals who work with older adults can identify strategies that might help their older clients develop wisdom characteristics. Problem-solving strategies, for example, might be amenable to counseling contexts where older clients are dealing with late-life concerns. Positive aging, therefore, may represent a kind of lifestyle, the consequence of which produces a "wisdom" skill set which can be used as a resource for adapting to the challenges of aging. The research seems to agree that possessing a "wisdom skill set" produces positive life outcomes.

In this regard, the connection between wisdom and well-being was examined in a study of 120 elderly people who were enrolled in the Berkeley Guidance Study, a large scale longitudinal investigation of adult development in the late 1960s. In this study, measures of life satisfaction and wisdom were obtained. Wisdom was operationalized as the capability of a person to integrate the cognitive, reflective, and affective components of problems or issues (Ardelt, 1997). Wise individuals were able to isolate the most important aspects of a life problem (cognitive), engage introspective skills when approaching such a problem (reflective), and understand the emotional aspects of a problem (affective). This study documented a strong relationship between those individuals who possessed wisdom and the ability of these persons to cultivate a sense of well-being irrespective of their living conditions. It was found that wisdom had a stronger influence on life satisfaction than socioeconomic status.

The ability to acquire wisdom in old age not only has a positive impact on those who encounter wise persons, but also means that older people who possess wisdom know how to age in a more satisfying way. Wisdom is linked to positive aging and coping mechanisms that are accessed through positive aging to maximize well-being and life satisfaction in old age are at the basis of cultivating a "wisdom skill set."

CONCLUDING COMMENTS

This chapter examined the nature and scope of age-related change with respect to several trajectories of decline descriptive of human aging. Normal aging was distinguished from successful and impaired/diseased aging due to their differential decline trajectories and the age-range confidence intervals at the point of death. The qualitative distinction between age-related and disease-related decline was explored as well as strategies (particularly memory strategies) from SOC for remediating age-related deficits. The final section of this chapter examined wisdom as a life skill that emerges for some people from years of experience. Wisdom was conceptualized as a form of knowledge or learning that is achieved as a result of learning from life's challenges and opportunities. Strategies for promoting wisdom in old age were presented, including how the effective application of SOC can cultivate wisdom in later life.

Chapter 4

ASSESSMENT STRATEGIES AND INSTRUMENTS

PROFESSIONALS WHO PROVIDE MENTAL health services to an older clientele should not only be skilled in distinguishing normal aging from disease, but should be able to address an older client's concerns by credibly evaluating the client's relative strengths and weaknesses. Standardized assessment tools should be part of every geriatric practitioner's evaluation and treatment repertoire, especially as these are employed to help gauge a person's present level of functioning across physical, emotional, and intellectual domains (American Psychological Association, 2004). An older client who is experiencing normative age-related deficits in any area of functioning may have legitimate concerns about his or her continued well-being. A pressing question in this instance is whether such deficits will get worse, continue on at essentially the same level, or gradually decline as one ages. In other words, the trajectory of an emergent deficit during the process of aging is important for an older client to know if the client hopes to cope. An in-depth examination of assessment instruments and strategies is beyond the scope of this chapter; however, the topic of assessment is addressed here to cover key areas related to assessment that are critical in promoting positive aging in later life. An evaluation of mood as well as a client's capacity for functional independence can provide important information about whether a disease is present as well as determine the extent to which enhanced quality of life is possible for a given elderly client.

One of the most common concerns an older person might initially present in counseling (and often the motivating reason for seeking counseling) is whether a noticeable cognitive problem or pattern of problems—such as forgetting the names of familiar persons—is simply a normal age-related deficit or signals the presence of a disease state such as AD.

The clinical picture of degenerative diseases such as AD can be very elusive, even for the trained clinician. As AD progresses, the long-term manifestations of profound cognitive deficits, including global memory impairment, inability to think abstractly, difficulty in understanding expressive language, and difficulty speaking fluently, all become markers of this deteriorative disease. It is also noteworthy, however, that if identified in its earlier stages, more can be done to remediate disease-related symptoms. Nevertheless, without sensitive assessment metrics, the disease can be mistaken for any number of issues that could be considered normative in old age. For this reason, it is essential that geriatric health care providers understand not only how to assess for age-related cognitive deficits, but how to distinguish cognitive problems due to normal aging from disease.

The Global Deterioration Scale (GDS; Reisberg, Ferris, de Leon, & Crook, 1982) is a widely accepted taxonomy for gauging cognitive deterioration due to AD. The stages of this scale are summarized in Table 4.1, which is based on Reisberg's published work (Reisburg, Ferris, de Leon, & Crook, 1988). Detailed behavioral manifestations that are descriptive of the behaviors at each stage can be found at (http://www.geriatric-resources.com/html/gds.html). AD severity on the GDS is measured on a 7-point range that is specifically related to change in cognitive functioning and functional ability associated with organic brain disease. Stages 1 and 2 are defined primarily by complaints (forgetting familiar names). Stages 3 and 4 are defined by observable deficits in functioning (reading a newspaper article and then being unable to remember what one just read, repeating a question over and over even though an answer has been given). Stages 5 through 7 are defined by the need for help or assistance in order to function in the everyday world (the need for assistance in balancing one's checkbook) and, in stages 6 and 7 help (or caregiver assistance) is absolutely necessary in order to address basic self-care needs such as bathing and eating. Without help, a person at a GDS, stage 7, would not survive.

A person who scored a 6 on this scale would suffer severe loss in functional capabilities needing continuing assistance to perform even the most basic tasks of daily living. Earlier in the process, when symptoms were at a GDS 4 or 5 a person still would have benefited from extended care placement (or services could have been initiated at home).

In many cases AD does not appear with full-blown symptomatology. Rather, its progression is often very subtle at first, and its early stages can be mistaken for many different normative age-related issues including old age forgetfulness, inattention, or absentmindedness. This is also true given that the course of AD is not always linear and there can be some temporary reversal of symptoms. Such symptom reversals can often be misperceived as the person finally coming back to his or her senses, when, in reality, it is only a mild fluctuation in the progressive pattern of deterioration. This turbulent pattern of symptoms can make AD very hard to evaluate without standardized assessment metrics.

It is often only when the behavioral manifestations of AD create clear functional deficits (spilling food on oneself while eating, getting

TABLE 4.1 GLOBAL DETERIORATION SCALE (GDS)

Stage	Description	Phase	Characteristics	Diagnosis
1	No decline	Normal	No complaints	Normal
2	Very mild decline	Forgetful	Complaints only	Minimal deficits
3	Mild decline	Mild confusional	Decreased performance	Suspect of AD
4	Moderate decline	Confusional	Clear-cut deficits	Mild AD
5	Moderately Severe decline	Early dementia	Needs help	Moderate AD
6	Severe decline	Middle dementia	Deficits even with help	Moderately severe AD
7	Very severe decline	Late dementia	Vegetative	Severe AD

*Note: The GDS is adapted from the published work of Reisberg et al., 1982 and 1988.

lost in one's garage, locking oneself in the bathroom) or put a person at risk for harm (burning one's hand on the stove, walking aimlessly into busy traffic) that it causes those in close relationships to the person to seek professional help.

Assessment, therefore, plays an important role in early detection not only of disease states such as AD, but also for other conditions of aging that tend to get worse over time and affect overall well-being. Such is the case when strength and agility is impaired due to an age-related disease state and simple eye–hand coordination necessary to perform functions, such as turning on a light, become impossible. The sections that follow focus on four areas of assessment that are germane to age-related decline and the emergence of disease: mental status, mood, adaptive functioning, and quality of life.

ASSESSING MENTAL STATUS IN OLDER ADULTS

Detecting and identifying change in general functional abilities can be challenging unless there are quality methods for assessing a person's overall intellectual functioning in the everyday world. This kind of functioning is commonly termed *mental status*. Geriatric health care practitioners employ standardized instruments that can assess functioning across a variety of intellectual abilities. The mental status examination is the format through which standardized information is obtained to determine whether a decline in functioning represents an impaired (or deficit) state, and, if so, what stage it has progressed to with respect to a normative group of similar aged adults. The mental status examination is the most important method of assessing general cognitive functioning in an older adult who may be complaining of difficulties with respect to intellectual or cognitive processes needed to negotiate tasks in everyday living.

In its basic form, a mental status examination is simply an objective description of a person's mental condition. This involves the coherence of a person's thoughts, mood, and behavior. Although several mental state examinations will be described in this chapter, it is important to note that the mental status exam is not limited to self-report questionnaires. In fact, the more comprehensive mental status examinations are often based on a person-to-person interview with a health-care professional or even a formal interview that involves the rating of prepared questions that systematically assess aspects of mental, physical, and emotional functioning. Most commonly, however, it usually includes a self- or other-completed questionnaire about the person's mental state. An excellent in-depth reference for assessing mental status in older adults can be found in *The Handbook of Assessment in Clinical Gerontology* (Lichtenberg, 1999).

There is high consistency in domains of functioning that are assessed by a mental status exam. Below are five areas that are essential to examine in order to assess mental state. Sample questions underscore how each area might be assessed:

- General orientation to time and place:
  Do you know what day it is today?
- The ability to hear and understand
  Can you pick up that pencil and put it on the table?
- Short- and long-term memory functioning
  Remember the word hat? *What am I wearing on my wrist?*
- The ability to engage higher intellectual abilities
  How are an orange and an apple similar?
- The ability to engage symbolic processes
  Can you write a sentence for me?

There are many conditions and situations in addition to aging that can affect mental status, including organic brain syndromes such as Alzheimer's disease (described earlier), psychiatric conditions (schizophrenia), traumatic events (a blow to the head), and extreme environments (high altitudes). Therefore, there are large numbers of mental status examination format options available to the practitioner with the type of exam designed for different contexts or clientele (children, adults, older adults). Below are several specific mental status examination questionnaires that are in general use with older populations. These instruments are readily available to the geriatric health-care practitioner. The Mini-Mental Status Examination and the Short Portable Mental Status Questionnaire are in the public domain.

The Mini-Mental Status Examination (MMSE)

The MMSE mental status examination questionnaire (Folstein, Folstein, & McHugh, 1975) was developed to quickly identify impairment in a number of different domains. This relatively simple paper-and-pencil instrument requires between 5 and 10 minutes to administer. There is a well-developed scoring scheme for the MMSE that ranges from 0 to 30 points with the higher scores indicating better mental status functioning. The MMSE covers several areas of functioning that are related to mental abilities (Hill & Bäckman, 1995). These domains are highlighted below:

- Orientation to place and time (*Where are you at right now?*)
- Attention (*Pick up this pencil and place it on the table*)
- Short and long-term memory (*Say three words and learn them for later recall*)
- Receptive and expressive language ability (*Read this sentence out loud to me*)
- Gross motor skills (*Fold this paper*)
- Spatial reasoning and functioning (*Draw a diagram*)

For the older adult who is in good health and is functioning adequately, obtaining a score of 30 on this instrument requires little effort. However, a number of validation studies with the MMSE have established cut-off scores; that is, errors in performance sufficient to warrant concern that a disease process might be present. A score under 25 on the MMSE signals that cognitive dysfunction is sufficient to warrant additional psychological testing to further elucidate the nature of the observed impairment (i.e., whether it is due to a disease process or some other problem such as a medication interaction). An MMSE score below 20 indicates that cognitive problems are present to a degree that is sufficient to impact aspects of daily living that involve mental functioning. A person scoring below 20 on the MMSE would have trouble negotiating even very simple everyday living tasks and would certainly be unable to live or function in contexts that demand higher-order cognitive skills.

The MMSE is an essential screening tool for the geriatric health care provider for several reasons. First, because it is, perhaps, the most widely used and generally accepted measure of cognitive status, most practitioners readily accept that a deficit score on the MMSE justifies additional diagnostic investigation (Tombaugh & McIntyre, 1992). Second, for a relatively brief instrument, the MMSE has excellent psychometric properties including good reliability and validity; that is, the MMSE tends to measure what it purports to measure (e.g., cognitive status) and an examinee's performance is relatively stable over time (Mitrushina & Satz, 1991). A measurable drop in MMSE score between administration intervals could be an indication that a disease process is present. It has also been used across a wide range of patient populations, so its applicability for most problems that involve cognitive deficits in old age including stroke, drug interactions, head trauma, dementia and other forms of organic brain syndromes, as well as disease-related cognitive deficits (cognitive problems associated with chronic obstructive pulmonary disease or heart disease) is strong (Cockrell & Folstein, 1988). The MMSE, however, is not without its problems including that it provides little information to guide specific remedial strategies. In addition, because MMSE scores are subject to floor and ceiling effects, it is not useful for distinguishing between subtle differences in cognitive performance in the early stages of AD (Anthony, LeResche, Niaz, von Korff, & Folstein, 1982).

The Dementia Rating Scale (DRS)

The Dementia Rating Scale (DRS; Mattis, 1989) is a more extensive mental status paper-and-pencil examination that involves 36 tasks and requires about 30 minutes to complete. Like the MMSE it covers specific areas of mental functioning, including attention, initiation and construction, conceptualization, and memory. The DRS also yields a composite score for an overall measure of mental status functionality. The DRS it provides multiple tests for each of the domains allowing more certainty about which particular mental abilities are problematic, and thus providing additional clues as to the nature and type of the problem. It also provides more information about what specific scores might mean in terms of mental deficits. The DRS has been used, for example, to identify different subtypes of dementia such as vascular dementia (Alexopoulos et al.,

1997), which would be difficult to pinpoint using the simpler MMSE score.

The DRS, however, does require more time and more skill to administer. For a practitioner who does not generally work with older individuals or is in a care context where most of the people do not have dementia or Alzheimer's disease, the DRS may be too involved and too difficult to use as a screening tool.

Another drawback to the DRS is that, unlike the MMSE, the DRS scoring keys and forms are not in the public domain, so it is necessary to purchase this instrument from an authorized test distributor. Finally, because it takes longer to administer, older patients may not be as willing or able to sit for the 30 minutes required to take the examination. In some instances, the DRS can be given over several days; however, this can reduce the reliability of the instrument because it does require standardized administration procedures.

The Short Portable Mental Status Questionnaire (SPMSQ)

Like the MMSE and the DRS, the SPMSQ queries an individual across several domains of functioning (Pfeiffer, 1975). Below are examples of questions from the SPMSQ:

- What is the: *day, month, and year?*
- What is the *day of the week?*
- What is the *name of this place?*
- What is your *phone number?*
- How *old are you?*
- When were you *born?*
- Who is the *current president?*
- What was you *mother's maiden name?*
- Can you *count backward from 20 by 3s?*

The SPMQ yields an error score from 0 to 10. The more errors made on these questions the greater the client's impairment. With respect to validated norms, 3 to 4 errors is indicative of mild impairment, a score greater than 4 errors indicates that impairment is unambiguously present. Scores of 3 or more would warrant additional psychological testing to determine the extent and nature of the mental status deficits. The SPMQ in itself is not able to provide much information about the nature of mental status deficits, but it does have several attributes that make it complementary to the MMSE or the DRS. Perhaps the most important is that because it requires only verbal responses to the questions, it is possible to administer this instrument over the phone (or even via the Internet) in order to determine whether a mental status problem might exist. For this reason, it is an ideal screening tool for the practitioner interested in working with larger numbers of older adults who are heterogeneous with respect to their independent functioning.

The three mental status examinations that have been reviewed in this section are typical of what the geriatric health-care practitioner might employ to assess the functioning of an older adult in a community context. There are many more like these that are available in the scientific and professional literature. However, it is important to note that this kind of examination format is not a replacement for a more comprehensive neurological evaluation when there is some indication that there may be a disease process present. In this case, a comprehensive examination may involve a medical exam including specialized laboratory testing, a brain scan, and a detailed clinical history of the individual to pinpoint the source and nature of the problem.

ASSESSING MOOD IN OLDER ADULTS

Older adults commonly complain about symptoms of anxiety and depression. Anxiety and depression can reduce emotional resources and make positive aging more difficult. Thus, it is important for the geriatric care provider not only to have the skill and tools to identify such symptoms, but also to be sensitive to the signs and symptoms of depressive or anxious affect and their linkage to adaptive functioning.

Depression

Depression is a prolonged state of low mood. Distinguishing features of a depressed state include a sense that life is hopeless, feelings of guilt, or the inability to experience pleasure. People diagnosed with clinical depression may have difficulty sleeping, eating, and performing tasks of everyday living. They may also talk about suicide or feel that the world would be better off if they were no longer alive.

Positive aging is not necessarily inconsistent with the situational experience of depression because most people experience aspects of low mood at various times during their life span. Depression can be triggered by a single traumatic event such as the diagnosis of a chronic illness, the loss of a long-term spouse, or change in living environment. Data suggest that when an older person loses a spouse to death, the likelihood of experiencing some symptoms of depressive affect is above 50% (Sable, 1991). When this occurs, it may be more difficult for a person in later life to rebound from the trauma of bereavement and begin to build a sense of well-being and satisfaction (Stroebe & Stroebe, 1987). Depression is also a risk factor in older persons suffering from chronic disease or in otherwise poor physical health. Because declines in physical health are highly likely in old and very old age, depression can be an emotional consequence of age-related physical decline (Berkman, Berkman, & Kasl, 1986). Finding ways to deal with situational depression in old age is a sign that a person is capable of positive aging, although one aspect of this may be some short-term treatment to address symptoms of depression and even the administration of medication to help the person compensate for low mood. In any case, it is important that assessment tools are available to identify depressive affect in order to engage strategies that can help to ameliorate it.

The Geriatric Depression Scale (GDS)

The GDS is a self-report measure of depressive symptoms in older adults. It was developed by researchers at Stanford University in the 1980s and since then has been substantially revised to make it more applicable to practitioners who work with older adults (Yesavage et al., 1983). The GDS assesses 15 areas that are related to depressive affect: satisfaction with life; change in activities; feelings of emptiness; feelings of boredom; level of mood; fear of the future; happiness; helplessness; getting out into the community; memory complaints; gratitude for being alive; worthlessness; energy level; hopelessness; comparing one's self to others.

There are a number of references that include the scale in its entirety as well as the scoring scheme (Yesavage, 1986). The GDS is an appealing instrument because its "true–false" format is simple and easy to administer. The GDS is also a very short 15-item paper-and-pencil measure, and the questions are worded so that they are relevant to older adults. It was specifically designed for the practitioner, but it has been used widely in research as well. In this regard, the scoring scheme is straightforward. Specifically, if a person endorses more than 5 of the 15 GDS questions in a negative way, such a frequency of response is suspicious of depression. Because it is not always possible to identify clinical depression using the GDS, it is important to remember that for those persons who score above 5 it is strongly recommended that they receive a more extensive evaluation of the nature of the depressive affect through an in-person diagnostic interview with a licensed mental health professional.

Like the GDS, The Cornell Scale of Depression in Dementia (CSDD; Alexopoulos, Abrams, Young, & Shamoian, 1988a) was designed to assess depression in older persons who may also have cognitive problems (including dementia). The 19-item CSDD addresses similar content areas to those items covered by the GDS. For the CSDD, the content areas include: sadness, inability to experience pleasant events, irritability, agitation, motor retardation, physical complaints, loss of interest, loss of appetite, weight loss, lack of energy, mood swings at different times during the day or night, difficulty falling asleep, waking up during sleep, waking up earlier than normal, suicidal thoughts, poor self-esteem, pessimism, and mood-related delusions. Unlike the GDS, the response format for the CSDD involves a 3-point ranking labeled as: (1) absent, (2) mild or intermittent, and (3) severe. Instead of endorsing an item as "yes or no" the CSDD evaluates whether there is evidence that a certain depressive symptom is absent, exists in a mild form, or is substantially observable. Higher scores on the CSDD reflect more depressive affect and a score of eight or greater indicates that depression is likely present.

The CSDD requires approximately 20 minutes to administer, which is somewhat longer than the GDS; however, the information for each question can be obtained either directly from the elderly examinee or from the caregiver (or corroborated by both). For this reason, it is a useful instrument to include, in addition to the GDS, if a care provider wants to determine whether symptoms of depression are confounded by cognitive impairment. When an elderly person is experiencing cognitive problems and depression, the reliability of the GDS may become somewhat suspect, particularly if there is a concern as to whether the elderly examinee understands a specific item. However, verification of one's affective state is possible when the CSDD is used. Research has shown that the CSDD is also effective in identifying depression in elderly persons who are cognitively intact (Alexopoulos, Abrams, Young, & Shamoian, 1988b).

Anxiety

Anxiety is an emotional state associated with a range of symptoms that include racing thoughts, a feeling of dread, agitation, and uneasiness. Anxiety and its symptoms can be a problem in old age. Even for a person who would not be diagnosed with an anxiety disorder, the situational experience of worry, restlessness, muscle tension, and sleep disturbance are ubiquitous issues that plague many people across the course of life. Like depression, stressors can catalyze symptoms of anxiety and, in late life, concerns about health, excessive worry about finances, the introduction of new people into the home as part of in-home care, or relocation when extended care is needed, could all be significant sources of situational anxiety. Unfortunately, because anxiety often creates physiological changes (e.g., fight or flight response to a stressor) it may not be sufficient that the trauma is resolved for symptoms of anxiety to go away. For this reason, anxiety could be a more widespread problem in old age than depression.

Anxiety Screening Tool

The assessment of anxiety in older adults is less straightforward when it comes to identifying a specific instrument or scale that measures anxious symptomatology. One of the challenges in this regard is that depressive symptoms overlap with anxiety symptoms to a great degree. Therefore, many depression screening measures such as the GDS described above contain items that also gauge anxiety. Other more general instruments, such as the Brief Symptom Inventory (Derogatis & Melisaratos, 1983), assess psychopathology in a more ubiquitous way and although anxiety subscales exist in such a measure, much of the information is irrelevant in otherwise healthy older adults. Goldberg, Bridges, Duncan-Jones, and Grayson

(1988) provided some guidelines to the practitioner who needs to gauge anxiety in an older person. From these items it is possible to develop an informal inventory to assess the symptomatic expression of anxiety. Like the GDS, these items could be organized in a true–false format for ease of administration. The specific items are listed below:

- Have you felt keyed up?
- Have you been worrying excessively?
- Have you been irritable?
- Have you had difficulty relaxing?
- Are you having difficulty sleeping?
- Are you having tension headaches?
- Do you feel nervous (trembling, sweating, heart palpitating)?
- Do you feel fearful about something or someone?

Endorsing five or more of these items could suggest that an individual may be dealing with anxiety.

A structured interview procedure that can identify anxiety disorders in older persons is the Schedule for Affective Disorders and Schizophrenia (SADS; Endicott & Spitzer, 1978). It employs a series of questions that highlight specific symptoms of anxiety (as these are differentiated from depression and other psychiatric disorders). Question content from the SADS used to identify anxiety includes: feeling fearful, unsettled, or on edge, as well as physical problems including poor sleeping, agitation, or a racing heartbeat. The SADS involves a 90-minute interview that provides a very reliable measure of anxiety, including its duration and severity. The SADS would be an appropriate measure to employ if an older person showed symptoms of anxiety on a shorter screening instrument and if the practitioner wanted more information about the nature and course of anxiety in such a patient.

Anxiety, like depression, is amenable to treatment; however, unless there is a way to gauge the extent to which a person is experiencing anxious symptoms it is difficult to develop meaningful strategies for treatment. In some instances support and reassurance may be the most effective approach, but in other cases, this palliative strategy may not address the underlying mechanism that is causing the problem. In this latter case, psychotherapy or pharmacotherapy may be important to consider as treatment options. It is then that a more comprehensive assessment procedure should be considered as a follow-up to the screening instruments described in this section. A comprehensive assessment would involve additional questions about the impact of anxious symptoms on mental status and everyday functioning. This would require a personal interview, including a physical examination.

Mood fluctuations across the life span are common. For many people, mood is influenced by life events, both positive and negative. Positive aging requires managing mood, and a first step toward effective management is recognizing when a person is experiencing a mood problem. The instruments above were selected from existing published scales because of their ease of administration, availability to the practitioner, and their relevance to older adults.

ASSESSING ADAPTIVE FUNCTIONING IN OLD AGE

Adaptive function has been traditionally defined as the extent to which a person can engage in everyday living tasks and personal self-care behaviors in order to function independently at home and in the community (Lawton & Brody, 1969). For many older adults, functioning independently for as long as possible is an important life goal. However, the longer a person lives the more likely it is that he or she will experience some form of age-related disability that makes independent functioning more difficult. It is important to be able to assess age related decline in functional independence.

Several studies note the association between chronological age and functional independence. These studies have documented that most people who are age 85 and older will have some form of age-related disability that will impair functioning (Hogan, Ebley, & Fung, 1999). Further, older persons who have difficulties carrying out daily activities are at higher risk for accidents that could lead to hospitalization or extended home care (Guralnik, Fried, & Salive, 1996). Therefore, assessing how well an older client can negotiate everyday living tasks is essential to helping him or her function independently for as long as possible.

The term *functional independence* (FI) has been used to describe an individual's capability to perform tasks essential to everyday living, particularly in older adults who are at risk for impairment, including the chronically ill, the frail elderly, and the disabled. In positive aging, the notion of functional independence does not imply the complete avoidance of assistance in everyday living, but focuses on the ability to determine, optimally, when help or assistance from another person is needed to maintain oneself independently. Several large-scale population-based studies, worldwide, have examined FI employing traditional measures of *activities of daily living* (ADL; Cutler, 2001; Bickenbach, Chatterji, Badley, & Ustun, 1999; Manton & Waidmann, 1998). In the form of paper-and-pencil surveys, ADL checklists assess ability to perform basic self-care tasks (such as bathing) with or without assistance from another person (Kane & Kane, 1981).

The Katz Adaptive Living Scale (ALS)

The Katz ALS scale measures functional independence through seven self-care activities: bathing, grooming, dressing, toileting, transferring from one place to another, continence, and feeding oneself (Katz, Downs, & Grotz, 1970). For these tasks, the older respondent (or a proxy) is required to report whether the older person who is being evaluated is able to perform these tasks: (1) without help, (2) with help, or (3) cannot perform the task even with assistance. As a marker of the progression of age-related disablement and the subsequent demand that a person's functional dependency places upon the support environment, accurately assessing ADL is critical for positive aging, particularly in very old age. The care implications, especially among those older adults who are already functionally limited, are essential to determine with respect to the costs and consequences of remaining functionally independent.

Only those individuals who can perform all seven activities on the Katz without needing help are rated as functionally independent. On the Katz Index, one point is assigned for each of the items where help is indicated. Two points are assigned for each item that cannot be performed even with help. Higher scores on the Katz indicate that a person is more functionally impaired.

It should be noted that with respect to dependency needs, the majority of older persons are not abruptly unable to engage in these kinds of self-care behaviors. Rather, there is often a gradual and natural progression of loss that manifests itself in problems that occur when someone is trying to negotiate a specific task. An older person who is at risk for loss of functional independence may go through several stages where the problem becomes worse. He may initially have trouble putting his shirt on and only need intermittent help fastening the buttons on his shirt. If this is progressive, over time this single difficulty may manifest itself in an inability to button trousers and shirt. The person could then lose the ability to put his shirt on. In this case, more help is needed. This help, then, would be the first objective indication that this individual was no longer functionally independent with regard to dressing himself.

Although this kind of issue might seem like a very minor problem, it would be an early sign that the ability to remain independent in a community context is going to become more difficult with the passage of time. The Katz is a very basic measure of this phenomenon. The weakness of the Katz is that a score is only obtainable if a person cannot negotiate a self-care task without help. The Katz would be of very little value as an assessment tool to measure the extent to which a self-care task is becoming more difficult to perform without help. For the older person who is able to perform these tasks alone, but only with great difficulty (versus the easy performance of such self-care tasks) other measures are needed to gauge ADL task difficulty.

The Gronigen Instrumental Activities of Daily Living Scale

For older adults who are at risk for loss of independence the development of more sensitive markers of functionality are needed to assess not only whether a person is functionally independent, but also whether there are early problems in functionality (Kempen, Miedema, Ormel, & Molenaar, 1996).

A more sensitive measure of functional independence should include a wider range of tasks such as those that involve getting along in daily life in addition to self-care items. This broader range of items might include household activities such as vacuuming, managing household finances, or doing the laundry. The inability to perform these tasks could also have consequences for functional independence. The term *instrumental activities of daily living* (IADL) has been used with respect to these kinds of complex independent living tasks that are critical for the individual's own living context within a community setting. The literature describing the measurement of IADL capability is less systematic than that available for ADL (Kane & Kane, 1981; Lawton & Brody, 1969); however, several commonalities between these two measures are noteworthy. First, both are focused on discrete tasks that are essential for independent functioning. Problems in functioning beyond these tasks are not directly assessed, although it could be inferred that the inability to perform a specific IADL task without help should be related to the broader range of activities not measured by IADLs.

Second, the metric of a more sensitive measure should evaluate not only whether a person could (or could not) engage in a task without assistance, but also how difficult it is for the person to perform this everyday living task. The Groningen Instrumental Activities of Daily Living Scale or GARS (Kempen et al., 1996) is an instrument that has both of these capabilities. The GARS was developed in the Netherlands, but it has been successfully used in the United States, France, Norway, and Sweden. It was developed for the express purpose of assessing functional impairment across ADL and IADL tasks. Thus, it is a longer and more involved instrument than the Katz. A strength of this instrument is that it can be assessed through a structured interview format or as a paper-and-pencil instrument that could be mailed to an older person. The GARS assesses both whether a person "can" perform selected activities as well as the extent to which a person feels "able" to perform ADL and IADL activities. The items on the GARS are: Can you dress yourself, get out of bed, stand up from sitting in a chair, wash your face and hands, wash and dry your whole body, get on and off the toilet, feed yourself, get around in the house (if necessary with a cane), go up and down the stairs, walk outdoors (if necessary with a cane), take care of your feet and toenails, prepare breakfast or lunch, prepare dinner, do light housework activities (dusting), do heavy housework activities (mopping), wash and iron your clothes, make the beds, shop?

Higher scores on the GARS indicate that a person is more functionally impaired. The designers of this instrument suggest that independent functioning is only possible if a person can engage in all of these 18 activities without help; however, different scores can be developed if there are contexts in which independent functioning is not required on a specific task. For example, if a person is living in a community where grocery delivery is part of the services provided, that task will not be a relevant measure of functional independence. The advantage of the GARS is that it covers a wider range of activities. This, however, is also a disadvantage in some cases where time is important and when there is resistance on the part of the older examinee to taking such an instrument.

Two independent living skills measures have been reviewed. Both are easily obtainable in the public domain and the Katz has been widely used in gauging the care needs of older adults. It is important to note that the issue of independent living becomes more pronounced the longer a person lives. It is also important to note that although disability is often viewed as irreversible, changing the context (where mobility is easier) or obtaining adjunctive supports (such as hearing aids, glasses, or a walking cane) can prolong functional independence and should be considered when assessing whether a person can function independently in old age.

The nature of age-related functional independence and positive aging are substantially interconnected; however, positive aging does not necessarily mean that a person is entirely independent. On the contrary, a positive ager is someone who is actively coping and developing strategies for compensating for functional decline as it occurs as a predictable part of the aging process.

ASSESSING QUALITY OF LIFE IN OLD AGE

Because age-related disability is progressive it is important that the geriatric practitioner is facile in the administration and interpretation of several instruments that are capable of measuring the full range of daily living issues from those that are manifest at the very earliest stage of disability (e.g., the ability to do the dishes without help or consistently misplacing one's belongings) to self-care issues that make it impossible for a person to remain in the home without some kind of ongoing assistance (e.g., the ability to toilet one's self). The research suggests that Instrumental Activities of Daily Living (IADL) diminish first, followed by more basic self-care behaviors that are characterized by ADL measures (Nourhashemi et al., 2001). Because preserving daily living skills for as long as possible is essential to prolonging positive aging, it is important to not only actively assess an older person's capabilities in this regard, but to have available techniques and strategies that a person can learn in order to adapt to age-related functional decline in these areas. Accurate assessment produces the highest likelihood that a suggested compensatory strategy will match the kinds of daily living problems that an individual is encountering at the point of assessment.

Assessing quality of life in old age is a complex undertaking. Not surprisingly, there are no generally accepted standards about how quality of life should be measured. Most of what we know about quality of life comes from research studies that have employed a wide range of research-based instruments to measure and define it. In many respects most studies of this nature are designed to answer more conceptual questions about the epistemology of quality of life and the nature of life satisfaction in old age. From a more practical perspective and one that has relevance for positive aging; however, it is critical that older people be able to enjoy who they are, what their living context is, and find happiness in the activities they are engaged in, as well as with those whom they interact. Positive agers are particularly in tune to these kind of needs and work very hard to address issues of quality of life as they age. So, in a sense, assessing quality of life requires attending to a broader set of needs in relation to personal circumstances. Assessment is critical in determining what is in the best interest of an older person who desires to preserve his or her quality of life for as long as possible, and this is especially true when persons are attempting to preserve quality of life in the presence of age-related decline.

It is also possible to assess quality of life through paper-and-pencil measures. Because this area of assessment does not have extensive applied research to draw from, it is not always possible to connect the items from an instrument used to measure quality of life and a model of care or counseling that is being used to promote quality of life in an older client. For this reason, the quality of life instruments described in this section relate to the models of adult development described in Chapter 2. These are, to some extent, more complex and multifaceted inventories; however, instruments that assess quality of life in this way can offer more insight into whether an individual can experience positive aging in late life.

The Selective Optimization and Compensation (SOC) Questionnaire

The SOC questionnaire is a 48-item scale developed by Paul Baltes and colleagues at the Max Planck Institute in Berlin, Germany (Baltes, Baltes, Freund, & Lang, 1999). The items address four areas of functioning that are descriptive of SOC; namely Elective Selection (ES): the ability to develop clear and specific goals in old age that are relevant to the individual and his or her context; Loss-Based Selection (LBS): the ability to focus only on the most strategic goals when faced with diminishing personal resources in old age; Optimization (O): the ability to redefine goals to make them achievable; Compensation (C): the ability to find ways to offset age-related deficits that are barriers to achieving goals (Baltes et al., 1999). A sample of paraphrased items from the SOC Questionnaire that describes each category is listed below:

- Elective Selection: I concentrate all my energy on a few things *or* I divide my energy among many things.
- Loss-Based Selection: If I can't do something as well as before, I concentrate only on essentials *or* Even if I can't do something as well as before, I pursue all my goals.
- Optimization: I keep trying until I succeed at a goal *or* I don't keep trying very long, when I don't succeed right away at a goal.
- Compensation: When it becomes harder for me to get the same results, I keep trying harder until I can do it as well as before *or* When it becomes harder for me to get the same results as I used to, it is time to let go of that expectation. (Baltes et al., 1995)

The SOC Questionnaire employs a fixed-choice response which requires the respondent to endorse one or the other option. It is scored by totaling the number of positive endorsements and negative endorsements. A higher positive score indicates a greater preference to utilize SOC strategies for life management. Those with higher positive scores on this instrument would be interpreted as being more adaptive to the changing nature of functioning in old age and more able to pursue goals consistent with one's life span trajectory. This kind of individual would be characterized as a positive ager.

Baltes and his colleagues have published several studies that have examined the usefulness of the SOC Questionnaire for predicting adaptability in old age. In one study, it was found that those who more strongly endorsed SOC strategies for life management were lower in psychopathology including neuroticism (Freund & Baltes, 2002). The SOC Questionnaire is a promising instrument that could link theoretical constructs of how to achieve well-being and adaptation through the application of life span management skills in old age to the emergence of counseling strategies designed to address the specific psychological needs of the older adult in this regard.

It has been used in cross-cultural studies that have examined the extent to which older persons have engaged positive aging in adapting to the challenges of age-related decline. In one study that evaluated the SOC Questionnaire in approximately 400 older Chinese adults (Chou & Chi, 2001) researchers examined not only its psychometric properties, but the extent to which it could measure well-being. The three SOC subscales were positively correlated with well-being and life satisfaction, and negatively correlated with depressive affect. Those individuals who engaged in positive self-management behaviors with respect to selection, optimization, and compensation tended to adapt better to challenges in late life and were less susceptible to psychiatric symptomatology including depressive affect. This finding suggests that SOC may have promise as a general measure of late-life adaptation across cultural groups.

The Satisfaction with Life Scale

The Satisfaction with Life Scale or SWLS (Pavot & Diener, 1993) is a brief self-report inventory consisting of five items: (1) In most ways, my life is close to ideal; (2) The conditions of my life are excellent; (3) I am satisfied with my life; (4) So far I have gotten the important things I want in my life; (5) If I could live my life over I would change almost nothing" (p. 172).

Each item represents one content domain that corresponds to a specific area of life satisfaction. The item response format is a 7-point scale anchored by strongly disagree (1) to strongly agree (7). The full text of the questions and a detailed description of the scale can be found in the research literature (Diener, Emmons, Larson, & Griffin 1985; Pavot & Diener, 1993). Although the SWLS has been used as a research tool, it also has application for assessing positive aging in cognitively intact older adults.

The SWLS scale is well suited to address issues of quality of life (Diener, 2000). As Pavot and Diener (1993) have noted: "The SWLS items are global rather than specific in nature allowing respondents to weight domains of their lives in terms of their own values, in arriving at a global judgment of life satisfaction" (p. 164).

The SWLS can also be used to determine quality of life in old age from within the continuity theory framework, namely: (1) The wording of the scale highlights its focus on the positive aspects of the older adult experience. When developing interventions' approaches for the older client, the strengths of the client should be at the forefront. This is opposed to the traditional approach to counseling that focuses only on ameliorating the weaknesses or deficits that the client may report. (2) Although there are only five questions in the SWLS, they are balanced with respect to focusing on the present and the past. Past experiences are evaluated for their influence on present functioning. Several items in the SWLS underscore this notion: item 5, "If I could live my life over again, I would change almost nothing" versus item 2, "The conditions of my life are excellent." The connection of the past to the present, with respect to coping strategies, is a central tenet of continuity theory. Therefore, positive aging is the experience that life can be viewed along a continuum of past-present-future and that coping strategies that worked in the past will be relevant in the future. (3) The scale is sensitive to the idea that life satisfaction is dependent upon the comparison of life circumstances to standard of living. The SWLS was developed with the notion that people, when they judge their own life situation tend to judge that quality of life as better (or worse) based on their own past experiences (not the current or past experiences of others). In this sense, the SWLS is based on the notion of stability among individuals over the passage of time and it is this sameness (or stability) that tends to be the focus of self-appraisal over time (Diener & Diener, 1996).

Although it is not easy to objectively assess quality of life in old age, it is very important to gauge the extent to which a person perceives that her or his life is "good" and has been satisfying in the past. Further, whether a person is able to experience quality of life may be related to how well he or she can develop coping resources to deal with the challenges of growing old. Again, positive aging does not require that a person be free from chronic disease or always experience high quality of life, only that the person can find hope and well-being through active coping with the challenges presented in life.

CONCLUDING COMMENTS

This chapter has examined assessment tools used to identify areas of deficit and strength in older persons with respect to mental status, mood, functionality, and life satisfaction. Specific instruments and the rationale for employing them in the assessment process are described. The geriatric health-care provider should have at his or her disposal a repertoire of instruments to guide interventions that can promote positive aging in later life.

Chapter 5

PSYCHOLOGICAL BARRIERS TO POSITIVE AGING

THE PERSONAL EXPERIENCE OF AGING is harder for some people than for others. In fact, some people have great difficulty growing old, not because their living context is objectively more difficult or harsh, but because they tend to make assumptions about themselves and their world that emphasizes the burdens of old age.

Personality theorists such as McCrae et al. (2000) and Costa and McCrae (1986, 1988) have argued that people are born with a set of selected predispositions, and it is the variation in these innate tendencies that accounts for the wide array of individual differences in personality in old age. Much of what we know about the makeup of personality across the life span comes from research that has investigated five personality traits of the five-factor model of personality. These are Neuroticism (N), Extraversion (E), Openness to Experience (O), Agreeableness (A), and Conscientiousness (C). A brief definition of these personality traits and an example that is descriptive of each dimension is summarized below (Costa & McCrae, 1986, 1992a, 1992b).

Neuroticism is descriptive of human pathology such as obsessive–compulsive thinking, dependency, and antisocial behavior. This trait is associated with a diminution in flexibility, the inability to take into account past history in making future decisions, and a restriction of psychological functioning. People who are characterized as neurotic have a hard time forming stable relationships, are indecisive in making important life decisions, tend to be anxious and fearful of the future, avoid responsibility, are prone to depression, worry excessively, and have the uncanny ability to place persons who care about them in the most difficult and conflicted life situations (Seidlitz, 2001).

Jim, age 59, described his adult life as unhappy. He had struggled to remain in relationships, but these had mostly ended badly. He had a very difficult time dealing with intimacy and the emotional flexibility required for maintaining long-term relationships. Although he was a talented draftsman, Jim had been unable to develop work habits to keep him consistently employed. Jim reported being very self-conscious at work and was prone to feeling anxious and depressed when given challenging job assignments.

Openness to Experience is a trait that is descriptive of flexibility in thinking and behaving. Openness to experiences underscores creativity and imaginativeness. People who are characterized by this personality dimension tend to be very independent minded and are able to think divergently or "out of the box." This kind of person is open to new ideas and looks for the novel aspects of living.

Susan was 63 and she described herself as a world traveler. She often said, "The world is my playground." What she enjoyed most about travel were the new sights and opportunities it afforded her to learn about culture and history. For most of her adult life, Susan was a high school teacher and she enjoyed teaching many subjects including math, reading, social studies, and anthropology. She was looking forward to developing a new unit in her curriculum about world cultures so that she could organize much of what she had learned in her travels into her advanced placement high school social studies course.

Extraversion is descriptive of an energetic approach to the social and material world and includes traits such as sociability, activity, assertiveness, and positive emotionality. People who are extraverted tend to be talkative, social, and assertive with others. They tend to portray not only gregariousness, but warm and positive emotions when engaging with other people. Extraverts tend to gravitate to careers that involve interacting with others in social and/or business pursuits.

> Sam was 72 and a sales representative for a farm implement store. He sold tractors to farmers. Sam had made a good living and could retire; however, he chose to stay employed because he continued to enjoy his work. He was proud of the fact that he frequently outsold the younger sales staff. He had a huge customer base and most of his days were spent driving out to farms and visiting with farmers and their work crews. This had built up a base of loyalty that was hard to match. When someone suggested that Sam retire his response was, "If I retired I would just continue to visit the same people, only I wouldn't make any money at it."

Agreeableness is a stylistic that emphasizes cooperation and a good natured attitude toward situations and others. People who score high on agreeableness have a propensity toward altruism. In group situations, a person who would score high on agreeableness may come across as tender hearted, although this kind of person is also capable of being very straightforward and fair in dealing with others.

> Sara was 77 and one of the central figures in her neighborhood. She was community service oriented and good to people. When neighbors had problems, she was the first to step in and help. Anyone who was around Sara felt included and cared about. She was a good listener and enjoyed letting people talk about themselves.

Conscientiousness is competence in thought and action. People who are conscientious tend to be self-disciplined and dutiful. They value orderly and dependable living as well as organized and productive working contexts. A highly conscientious person is one who is responsible and can be counted on to complete any task assigned to him or her. A conscientous person defines her or himself on indices of personal accountability and reliability.

> John, age 74, had been a mechanic for most of his life. He developed a reputation over the years as an excellent repairman

to bring automobiles to for service. His automobile repair business received several awards from the Chamber of Commerce for its high quality work. After John retired he began to focus more on his gunsmith hobby and started a small business out of his own home repairing and refurbishing guns. He became highly expert at gunsmithing and developed an extensive collection of guns that showed off his workmanship.

Specific self-report inventories have been developed that assess how people range on each of these domains. The Neuroticism, Extraversion, Openness to Experience Personality Inventory (NEO-PI, Revised; Costa & McCrae, 1992b) is a 181-item paper-and-pencil measure that is based on this five-factor model of personality. It requires the respondent to answer questions along a 5-point likert-type scale that ranges from (1) strongly disagree to (5) strongly agree. In addition to gauging where a person scores on each of the dimensions noted above, it also provides a profile of an individual with respect to his or her overall personality disposition, because it is assumed that there is substantial interaction among these personality traits in how a person construes her or his worldview. In clinical assessment, knowing an older client's NEO-PI profile can help the practitioner better understand the client's inner world, especially with respect to the client's emotional state, intra- and interpersonal style, and personal motivations.

A series of research studies has inquired as to whether an individual's personality disposition can predict objective behavior. In one such study involving 418 older volunteers, researchers attempted to determine whether the five-factor model of personality could predict a range of behaviors (Paunonen, 2003). The NEO-PI was administered to each participant along with an extensive self-report form to document whether they engaged in health risk or beneficial behaviors including tobacco and alcohol consumption, reckless driving behavior, dieting, buying lottery tickets, or donating blood. The findings were as hypothesized; personality did predict many of the behaviors noted above. In general, the nature of the relationship between personality and behavior was that when a person's NEO-PI score was in the negative or more maladaptive direction (higher neuroticism), the person was more likely to adopt behaviors that would put their health or psychological well-being at risk. Heavier alcohol consumption was related to lower conscientiousness and tobacco consumption was related to low agreeableness. This research suggests that it is possible to gauge how a person will act if you know the basic makeup of his or her personality.

Just as personality has been found to predict behavior, it has also been associated with one's sense of well-being. In one study, the NEO-PI predicted happiness in a sample of college students. Specifically, those scoring higher on the extraversion scale reported a higher degree of subjective well-being than those scoring low in extraversion (Pavot, Diener, & Fujita, 1990). In a related study that included 109 older women volunteers (average age 72.6 years), the five-factor personality model also predicted life satisfaction. Specifically, the neuroticism scale from the NEO-PI was found to be associated with a more positive overall sense of well-being; that is, those scoring lower on neuroticism (or less neurotic) reported less psychological distress and higher levels of life satisfaction (Boland & Cappeliez, 1997). Most studies that have been interested in the linkage between subjective well-being and the five-factor model of personality have concluded that the dimensions of neuroticism (less is better) and extraversion (more is better) are the most strongly associated with subjective well-being in old age.

For the mental health practitioner working with older persons, the acknowledgment of intrapsychic traits that by strict definition are not modifiable over time can represent a challenge to counseling and a barrier to positive aging. An extravert will always be an extravert no matter how much difficulty this personality trait creates for the person. What may be more productive to focus on in counseling are the behavioral manifestations of personality; that is, specific maladaptive stylistics that are more or less under a person's conscious control.

A maladaptive stylistic is a generic label that provides a practical way to identify beliefs or assumptions that a person chooses to make that can cause him or her to experience an emotionally negative burden. The burden may exist, not because reality is pressing on the person in any harmful or disarming way, but because this errant construal of oneself and others tends to produce a set of negative anticipatory emotions such as fear, panic, anger, or dread that one might justifiably feel in objective circumstances when a bona fide negative event has occurred. In many respects, because maladaptive stylistics are under conscious control, they are more amenable to change.

Although there is not a comprehensive taxonomy that can be used to characterize every maladaptive stylistic, the clinical literature has highlighted five that are summarized in the next section. These are rigidity, negativity, worry, self-absorption, and regret. In addition to a summary of these maladaptive stylistics, a case example of how these might be manifested in old age is presented along with a set of specific strategies that could be employed by a counselor, or as a self-help strategy to address the negative consequences of such a maladaptive stylistic and to challenge the underlying assumptions that result from the stylistic.

RIGIDITY

There have been a number of references to rigidity in the psychotherapy and counseling literature that have labeled it as a worldview inconsistent with healthy adaptation. Albert Ellis (1987) asserted that rigidity was one of the major barriers to good mental health because it prevented people from discarding irrational and maladaptive beliefs about themselves and their world. In the counseling literature, rigidity has been defined as a form of resistance to change, even when there is clear evidence that change will improve well-being or lead to healthier functioning (Mahalik, Cournoyer, DeFranc, Cherry, & Napolitano, 1998). It has also been suggested that rigidity represents a superficial way of thinking about problems and issues that does not benefit from deeper insights or reflection about solutions (Schultz and Searleman 2002). It is this latter definition that makes rigidity a maladaptive stylistic in old age. It does appear that as people age some become less flexible in their attitudes and behaviors (Botwinick, 1966; 1969; Schaie, 2005). The following example highlights the persistent nature of rigidity as an aspect of highly practiced habitual behavior: "Consider the case of a U.S. automobile driver who travels to England where it is customary to drive on the left side of the road. If, after several driving excursions, the driver is still unable (or unwilling) to adapt to the new prevailing rules of the road, then this would reflect rigidity" (Schultz & Searleman 2002, p. 170).

In old age, rigidity can be problematic in coping when it underscores a view of the world that is (1) narrow in focus and (2) not amenable to change either as a result of one's own process of introspection or due to feedback from others. It is a way of thinking and relating to others (and the world at large) that encompasses the tendency to be locked into static mental and behavioral sets (Schultz & Searleman, 2002). Rigid people assume that the world conforms to a specific order and that structure must be enforced on any form of ambiguity. The stronger this assumption, the more rigid a person's behavior becomes, and the more uncomfortable a person will feel in ambiguous contexts.

A rigid stylistic represents a barrier to positive aging for the following reasons: (1) It limits one's ability to see a problem from different perspectives as well as the capacity to consider multiple "options" for solving problems that might be encountered across the life span and in later life (such as age-related decline in functional mobility). (2) A person who adopts a rigid approach to problem solving is also likely to repeat a previously used strategy to solve a new problem, even if this flawed strategy did not work in the past. In essence, rigidity fosters repeating the same mistake twice.

The case example below highlights how rigidity might manifest itself in an older person's approach to solving a typical problem.

Bill, a retired insurance agent, was a widower who lived alone in his five-bedroom home. Bill had lived in this home for most of his adult life. Seven years earlier Bill's wife had died of cancer. This was a difficult loss for Bill, although he had strong support from his children as well as from his living siblings. When Bill turned 80, he noticed that his stamina and health seemed to be declining. He was unwilling to see his doctor about this health change because, in his view, "I don't want the doctor to tell me that I need to move out of my house." Bill's condition continued to deteriorate and he began to have symptoms of nausea most mornings. During a recent summer afternoon, Bill was alone on his patio when he experienced a profound dizzy spell which caused him to fall, hitting his head on the cement patio floor. He was unconscious for several hours until he was discovered by one of his children. Bill was rushed to the hospital and treated for a concussion. However, from a routine blood test, the doctor discovered that he had an advanced form of liver cancer and was terminally ill. Bill's children, upon learning the news, felt that they should have forced their father to get regular medical checkups, but realized that this would have been futile given their father's stubborn avoidance of doctors and the medical establishment.

This example highlights the consequences of Bill's rigid assumption about getting preventive medical checkups. Interestingly, although rigidity has not been strictly linked to the aging process, it is not uncommon for people to focus on the elderly man or woman who refuses to change his or her behavior or relinquish a point of view in spite of clear evidence that there are "better" or more "flexible" ways of behaving and thinking about such situations.

With respect to other features of aging that might appear to indicate rigidity, but are, in actuality, age-appropriate manifestations of positive aging, two aspects of aging factor in. First is the notion of behavioral (and cognitive) slowing as an objective consequence of normative age-related decline (Schaie, Dutta, & Willis, 1991). This phenomenon occurs for all people and is progressive with advancing age. So, it is important not to mistake rigidity (or the inability to think and relate flexibly to the world) and the speed of a specific response; that is, slower is not necessarily more rigid. The second confounding feature is the notion of cautiousness, which has received some attention in the scientific literature as a motivational force in old age (Botwinick, 1966, 1969; Yong, Gibson, de L. Horne, & Helme, 2001). It is evident from this literature that cautiousness may increase with advanced age (Yong et al.). However, in cautiousness, the overriding behavior is a more careful, reflective stylistic. Cautiousness is adaptive in old age and it should not be confused with the stubbornly inflexible behavior that is characteristic of a rigid assumption system. In the example above, the consequence of Bill's inflexibility about seeing a physician and getting a medical checkup had a negative consequence on his health. A cautious person, upon reflecting over a negative health change, would likely feel the need to check out this issue through appropriate medical means, especially if it had begun to cause discomfort or impair daily function. Bill's quality of life may have improved if he had pursued a more cautious approach by visiting his doctor to determine if his physical symptoms were signalling a medical condition needing treatment.

Strategies for Changing Rigidity

Although rigidity, for some, may be an ingrained lifestyle orientation, it is possible to help older persons learn ways of modifying this stylistic. Counseling could engage a few simple strategies for challenging a rigid lifestyle pattern, and in the process, help an older person build more flexibility into how he or she responds to the world. Below are several concrete suggestions in this regard:

- Consider other options before responding:
  Think before you act.
  Anticipate an outcome prior to taking an action.
- Examine your beliefs underlying tenets:
  Are they based on your own idiosyncratic thinking?
  Are they shared by at least a few other people?
  Are they sound with respect to what you know about the issue?
- Practice doing routine tasks differently:
  Take a different route to work.
  Act in a different way in a common situation (say hello to a passerby).
- Seek out new experiences in life and leisure:
  Go somewhere different on vacation.
  Eat at a different restaurant.
  Join a new club or group.
- Find ways to change who you are in meaningful ways:
  If you are overweight, join a weight-loss group.
  Challenge your personal assumptions about your world.
  Take a different position about a political or personal issue than you really believe just to practice presenting an alternative point of view.

These ideas are not presented as definitive strategies for counseling. They only represent examples that might encourage flexibility in thinking and acting that rigid people do not easily actualize. When challenging rigidity one key is to examine how and why it is important to defend or repeat a static position even if it is not adaptive or contributing to one's well-being. An important question to pose to a rigid client might be: Do you continue to engage in the same routine of thinking, feeling, and acting only because it is easier than changing?

Behaving in ways that show flexibility and examining one's thinking processes about rigidity is not easy at any age. The essence of this difficulty might be captured by considering that if one were standing in a long grocery line and, just before reaching the checkout, chose to step out of the line and return to the end, such a behavior could show flexibility. However, most people would resist doing this, nor would it appear, on the surface, to be very adaptive. If, however, the goal was to train oneself to be more flexible, it could be a demonstration that one's assumptions and habit-driven behavior can be altered if placed under conscious control.

NEGATIVITY

Negativity is a way of approaching the world that (1) is pessimistic and (2) assumes that whatever happens, it will somehow take away from one's well-being or life satisfaction. Negativity has also been termed *pessimism,* and in this regard has been defined in the scientific literature as a negative mindset or expectation about the future (Scheier, Carver, & Bridges 2001). Negativity relates not only to the future, but also how one appraises the past and present. In a sense, negativity is a kind of selective or biased attention to information or events that fit a specific belief profile. If an older person holds a negative point of view, then thinking about the past, the present, or future will always have a defeatist overlay. Negativity in old age, like rigidity, is a practiced maladaptive stylistic that, by virtue of choosing to identify and focus on the negative, is strengthened while at the same time the ability to be affirmative diminishes. Negativity is present in older persons who hold pessimistic views of themselves by choosing to selectively attend to information that is consistent with this worldview (Bem, 1970). Negativity can be at the root of why an older adult may feel distressed when he or she is reminiscing about the past, for example, "I never really loved my husband when he was alive."

A negative appraisal about one's past, present, and future presents a serious barrier to positive aging because: (1) It colors how one views people and situations in a way that distances the person from her or his sense of emotional well-being; that is, it makes it difficult for something that is viewed with negativity to also be perceived as having a positive valence ("My husband has his faults, but he is a good father when it comes to children"). This is a particularly important point because almost all events (and people) in life are not 100% positive or negative. (2) A person who is primarily negative about him- or herself and the world becomes harder to approach relationally. (3) Negativity creates a sense of impotence. When bad things inevitably happen, such events work to confirm that nothing can be done to change one's situation.

The case example below highlights how negativity might manifest itself in an older person's approach to solving a typical problem encountered in late life.

Carl, a retired 74-year-old geologist, had problems all of his life due to a negative attitude. Carl was in a 40-year marriage, although neither he nor his spouse would construe their marriage as happy. On his wife's account, she noted, "Carl and I stay together for our children, for the extended family, and for the Church." Carl had worked a number of jobs over his lifetime and most had ended badly with Carl either resigning or losing his job for ambiguous reasons. His last job as a staff geologist for the state Bureau of Land Management was, in his opinion, tolerable because as Carl noted, "The State paid me poorly but they left me alone to do the work I was assigned to do although it would have been nice to have had more 'honest' contact with my coworkers." Carl had few friends, although he did have a supportive family. His older brother, Richard, confronted Carl on several occasions about his negative attitude and told him, "Carl, I want you to say one good thing about yourself every day." Carl's response to this was, "Richard, you will need to write these good things down for me, because I surely won't be able to think of any or remember them."

Carl's negativity highlights the qualitative nature of a life colored by the lens of pessimism. Carl's story conveys the message that a negative attitude, if practiced over the life span tends to proliferate into all areas of a person's day-to-day experiences. In Carl's case, because he consistently and obsessively voiced negativity, it was very difficult for even his closest relations to interact with him in meaningful ways. One issue that is unique to aging, therefore, is the consequence of a long-standing pattern of negativity; that is, the longer it goes on the worse it may become.

Other features of aging might appear as negativity, but are, in actuality, from another source and may be an older person's objective view of the challenges and difficulties of old age. In a qualitative study that explored the meaning of suffering in old age (Black & Rubinstein, 2004), one theme emerged: [they found] "Many elders experienced suffering as transformative (p. 17) . . . that suffering was an event or state of being that altered their self-view and worldview in a fundamental way" (p. 23).

Suffering, like other forms of negative life experiences that face an older person, is a challenge from the external world to one's internal sense of continuity. Suffering, like grief, sadness, and pain, represents observable manifestations of persons coping with negative life conditions. Suffering can produce meaningful outcomes in terms of perspective, learning, compassion, change, and ultimately, increased maturity. So, when a person is experiencing a negative state of mind, it may be that this emerges from a phenomenon quite different from negativity or pessimism. More concretely, negativity comes from one's intrapsychic world as a way to shape the external environment and displace fear ("If I'm negative about something it can't hurt me"). Therefore, an essential difference between negativity and suffering is that suffering promotes greater meaning and understanding about one's life situation while negativity only offers escape from realistically dealing with a specific challenge or issue.

Strategies for Challenging Negativity

Although changing a negative orientation may, for some, seem very difficult, it has been possible for people to cultivate a more positive outlook on life by engaging in focused reframing strategies that are part of cognitive behavior therapies (Coon, Rider, Gallagher-Thompson, Thompson, 1999). It should be remembered that because a consistently negative person can be difficult to interact with, any positive statement that comes from someone who is engaged in a negative spiral will often be quickly noticed and heavily rewarded, particularly by those who are part of a negative client's social support network. Below are several ideas for challenging negativity.

1. The client can be challenged to keep track of his or her statements: If they are mostly negative some can be changed. Suggest the client start with one or two positive statements and observe the consequences when people hear them. Which statements really reflect an unchangeable situation and which are changeable (bad weather always gets better with time)?
2. Ask others around you for their feedback: Are you perceived as portraying negativity? Find positive statements to say about those you care about. Replace a negative thought with a positive statement.
3. Seek out experiences that are mostly positive: Engage in a pleasurable activity and overstate its positive nature.
4. Identify someone who is optimistic and follow their lead: What are the consequences of this person's optimistic worldview? How does this person maintain optimism even in difficult times?

The goal in transforming negativity is not to change one's entire set of assumptions about the world, but to begin practicing an alternative way of thinking and relating that is not always negative. One of the most important suggestions is to identify someone who has an optimistic worldview. By observing this person, one can discover the benefits from engaging in positive thinking about one's self, others, and the world.

WORRY

Worry is a form of mental preoccupation that can, in some instances, be a reasonable strategy a person engages in to deal with a potentially stressful life event. In this instance, worry might catalyze one's preparation for dealing with a future challenge or threat. For this reason, worry can be adaptive. In fact, many older adults have valid "life events" about which to worry. Worrying about a family member who is in a situational crisis or worrying about one's health if one is sick, can have a meaningful consequence for adaptation. However, worrying can consume time and emotional energy if it goes on excessively. A person who worries in excess about trivial issues or things that "are not worth worrying about" can suffer needlessly. When a person spends too much time worrying it can have serious negative psychological repercussions including depressive affect (Ruscio, Borkovec, & Ruscio 2003). It is this incessant pattern of worry that can be a barrier to positive aging.

In the scientific literature, there has been interest in measuring maladaptive worry in older adults. Below are items from the Revised Penn State Worry Scale that are specifically written to measure abnormal worrying in late life elders (Hopko et al., 2003). These items are useful as a way to better understand the qualitative nature of worry as a maladaptive stylistic.

- My worries overwhelm me.
- Many situations make me worry.
- I know I should not worry about things, but I just cannot help it.
- When I am under pressure, I worry a lot.
- I am always worrying about something.
- As soon as I finish one task, I start to worry about everything else I must do.
- I have been a worrier all my life.
- I have been worrying about things.

As highlighted in these items, when worrying is frequent and the intensity of worry is high it can pose a substantial barrier to positive aging for several reasons: (1) Worrying can be a negative experience that can influence other aspects of life that are a source of happiness and pleasure. When a person is preoccupied with worrying, nothing else seems to matter. (2) People can become overly sensitive to worrying about the smallest things. For example, physical aches and pains are part of becoming old and although some can be attenuated others will remain. Worrying needlessly about those aches and pains can lead to a narrowing of focus on life's difficulties even when it is not possible to do much about them. (3) Although not unique to older adults, worry about the past is often perceived as contributing to misery in old age. For example, a widow spent an inordinate amount of time worrying about the fact that the day before her husband died suddenly of a stroke, they had been in a disagreement about where they wanted to spend their next vacation. This was such a source of worry that it created health problems in the surviving widow years later.

The case example below highlights how worry might manifest itself in an older person's approach to solving a typical problem encountered in late life.

Doug is a retired social worker. He lives alone and has never been married. At 71 Doug was diagnosed with a curable form of skin cancer and is being treated for this by his doctor. Doug is very preoccupied with his health problem. He is very vigilant about when he goes outside, what he wears, and who he comes in contact with. He loses sleep at night thinking about his cancer, and most of the time he spends interacting with family members, including his ailing mother who is 97 years old, the topic of conversation is his cancer and concerns about his deteriorating health. Some of his long-standing friends have become more distant because Doug has been unable to meet with them, fearing that this might somehow affect his health condition. Doug wants, more than anything in the world, to be free from the debilitating concern about his cancer.

This example highlights the kind of preoccupation that is possible when one is unable to put a check on worrying. In many ways, Bill is probably not aware of the extent to which he is worrying because it is such an ingrained part of his everyday lifestyle. However, he is certainly aware of the acute emotional pain that this worry is causing him. In Doug's case, his worry is focused on himself and it is unrelenting.

Worry is a difficult maladaptive stylistic because most people worry about something from time to time across the course of living. And, in some cases worry is useful in that it can keep in awareness a task or an act that needs to be engaged in to deal with a stressful life event. However, the controllability of worry becomes harder when one cannot stop this process. Finding ways to manage worry is one key to experiencing positive aging.

Strategies for Managing Worry

Below are several strategies for managing excessive worry. The important issue here is learning how to worry about those things "worth worrying over" while at the same time not worrying about the things that do not need this level of emotional attention. This can be difficult in old age because there are a number of anticipated events that are legitimate sources of worry, including one's own health, the health of family members, financial security, and changes in functional independence and dying.

1. Make a list of your worries. Rank these items in terms of their seriousness. Select one item and move it from your worry list.
2. Examine your motivation to worry. Is this something that will appreciably affect your life and well-being? What are the consequences if your worries come true?
3. Practice finding other emotional reactions to a worry situation. Find ways to diffuse your worries. Learn to laugh at some of your worries.
4. Carefully examine those events from the past that continue to be sources of worry. What continues to fuel worry about a past event? Will worrying about this event change the nature of the present?

It is easy for a negative emotion like worry to dominate one's thoughts, feelings, and actions. In most instances, worry makes a problem bigger even if the objective nature of the problem does not change. However, with practice and conscientious effort, worry can be managed as part of an optimally adapted lifestyle; that is, worry can signal when emotional resources are needed but it does not have to be a needlessly preoccupying emotion.

SELF-ABSORPTION

The nature of self-absorption in old age is complex. The clinical literature is direct in pointing to the maladaptive quality of self-centeredness as it relates to coping and subjective well-being in adulthood. In fact, across the life course, as described in Erikson's model of life span development, one of the implicit outcomes of maturation is for the individual to move from a self-centered, self-absorbed perspective (as is apparent in early childhood) to a perspective that focuses on others. Recall from Chapter 3 that the seventh stage of Erikson's developmental model is generativity vs. self-absorption. The central importance of this stage of development, is learning deeper skills and knowledge about the uncertainties of living and then being able to pass this knowledge and learning along to others. Wisdom is a cognitive style that is other focused. People who fail to develop wisdom-related qualities in old age because of a self-absorbed stylistic will have a difficult time experiencing positive aging.

Self-absorption can take many forms, although a common manifestation is for a person to focus on him- or herself with respect to prioritizing the meeting of personal needs including desires, appetites, and preferences (to the exclusion of others). To do this one must construe him- or herself in a specific light. Raimy (1975) suggested that this kind of self-focus bias in perception might take two general forms: (1) I am special, or (2) something is wrong with me. These two aspects of self-absorption interact with the aging process in a number of ways. First, older adults can sometimes feel "entitled" with respect to themselves and others in their social world. Entitlement is a self-absorbed ideology that emphasizes the importance of one's specialness. The expectation that one "should" be cared for is a kind of thinking that places a barrier between the older adult and his or her potential caregivers.

The second misconception that "something is wrong with me" is predictably associated in old age with diminished function and increased vulnerability to disease and disability. The older adult who is self-absorbed with such present-focused pains and problems is often unwilling to believe that the end of aging is death. The acceptance of this fact is the final stage of Erikson's developmental model (integrity vs. despair). It is critical that one begin to let go of self-absorbed ideologies in order to meet the final life challenge of living which is one's own personal experience with death. A person who is hindered by a self-absorbed stylistic will tend to focus on the present. He or she will be unable to suspend this perspective in order to find a general sense of meaning and well-being in a life that has been fully lived.

The case example below highlights how self-absorption might manifest itself in an older person's approach to solving a typical problem in later life.

John is 87 years old. He has been widowed for five years. After his wife died he experienced difficulty adjusting because his wife had essentially been his domestic caregiver. Following her death, John's own health deteriorated and over a five-year period he spent very little time outside his home. When his children visited, John spent most of their time together complaining about his physical symptoms and expressing concerns about his health. His interest in his grandchildren was minimal. He noted, "I know I am going to die someday but I just can't accept this fact." John is not a hypochondriac or an excessive worrier in general, but he is interested in cures and anti-aging techniques that he sees on TV. He often orders these, tries them for a while, and then discards them. He feels unappreciated by his children and grandchildren. When they provide assistance to him he emphasizes the burden he is on the family. Recently, John broke a hip in a fall that occurred in his home. His children thought that he should move out of his house and live with one of them, but no one was willing to put up with John's persistent complaining and lack of appreciation for their efforts to help him. The oldest daughter said, "I'm willing to take Dad in, but he would constantly run me down. . . . I'm not sure I could be his substitute wife and caregiver. It would be hard to put up with his constant need for reassurance."

This example highlights the kind of behavior that a self-absorbed person might engage in. John has insight that his life will not last forever and that he will experience age-related decline, but he refuses (or is unable) to see the world from another person's perspective. For this reason he is not easy to approach relationally. He may have found some solace earlier in his life from his wife, who was most likely completely devoted to him, and probably reinforced John's sense of his own specialness at the expense of meeting her needs. From his children's perspective, John's verbal self-focused behavior makes him difficult to deal with and they feel conflicted when visiting him. John's lack of interest in their lives and his inability to appreciate their efforts to help him or include him in their family activities prevents them from assisting him, even when John is experiencing a pressing health need.

John is not happy with his life and he will likely never be happy unless he can find a way to divert some of his attention from his own needs and direct it toward others. It will be difficult for John to experience positive aging if he is unable to alter this self-absorbed stylistic.

Strategies for Reducing Self-Absorption

Self-absorption is difficult to change because it becomes, in and of itself, a source of meaning and purpose for living. From an adaptive point of view, focusing on oneself is essential if change is to occur. In this sense, however, that focus is more introspective, with the goal of identifying patterns or characteristics of one's own behavior that are amenable to change. Below are a few suggestions that might help a person begin to engage in an other-focused perspective. These suggestions could be a component of a more general counseling approach to help a self-absorbed older person find meaning in life.

1. Take notice of others in his or her social world, such as with family and friends. What is it about the client that allows him or her to maintain these relationships? Develop a curiosity about these people.

2. Examine the nature of the client's complaints. What do the complaints tell the client about him- or herself? Help the client learn to inhibit verbalizing those complaints.

3. Practice being grateful. Find things that the client can be grateful for in others. Encourage the client to express that gratitude, occasionally, to others.

4. Get the client to find a way to involve others in his or her lifestyle. Show positive affection for a loved one. Listen to others talk about themselves before reciprocating.

These general suggestions should not be construed as a comprehensive intervention approach, rather as a way to provide the client with some insight into the nature of her or his own self-absorbed state. This can be a challenging counseling process because often one of the features that maintains self-absorption is insularity from personal introspection. A second challenge to relinquishing self-absorption is that one must be willing to subordinate or subjugate one's personal needs and desires to those of others. This may seem, at one level, to diminish quality of life; however, if sincerely attempted it may instill new psychological realities, such as altruistic thinking, which has been found to enhance or build quality of life, even in the presence of difficult personal circumstances (Dulin et al., 2001).

REGRET

Regret is a negative stylistic that is often tied to an experience or set of experiences that have occurred in the past. In this regard, regret is one of those assumptions about life that is tightly linked to the aging experience, particularly because regret requires that a previous experience has occurred. Thus, because aging is the accumulation of more life experiences, growing old can be associated with an increase in the frequency of regrets.

As a formal psychological term, *regret* is commonly experienced when a person has an emotional attachment to some negative aspect of a previous experience that he or she has been a part of (Landman, 1987). Usually, when regret occurs, there is a judgment that a person makes about his or her role in that experience ("If only I would have said something nice to that person, he or she would not be so hard to talk with now"). Interestingly, some researchers have argued that there is a qualitatively different emotional experience when a person has regret for an action that has been engaged in ("I spoke harshly to my mother") versus not acting when an action was called for ("I should have stopped my car and helped that poor woman cross the street" (Seta, McElroy, & Seta, 2001).

Some scholars believe that regret may tend to exaggerate or distort the aspects of an objective event in a negative direction. When this happens, regret can sap emotional resources for dealing with present realities or for planning the future. The stylistic of regret emotionally freezes a person in the past at a single point in time (Lecci, Okun, & Karoly, 1994).

The emotional experience of regret includes feelings of despair, helplessness, sorrow, and often a sense of hopelessness about one's inability to change the nature of the regrettable event. When regret is intense, there can even be desperate emotions that are akin to anxiety and depressive symptoms as well as catastrophizing about the consequences of an historical event. In many ways, although regret is a ubiquitous phenomenon in our social world, its primary value is in preventing future mistakes. If you regret an action you may not do it again in the future. However, in many instances when a person experiences substantial regret, there is little adaptive value to it, particularly if it restricts the person to his or her past. Regret is almost always focused on the self and what one did or did not do. This is highlighted in the example below:

> Kevin, an 73-year-old alcoholic, lives in a halfway house with a dozen other men. He describes his life as a series of one problem after another filled with bad decision making and impulsive acts. He is currently divorced. He reports that his struggle with alcohol began in his adult years as he was trying to cope with a relatively difficult marriage. He says, "I regret ever having tasted alcohol." Kevin didn't think too much about the future because he feared that if he became more independent he would become impulsive, start drinking again, and ultimately end up worse off than he was currently. He spent most of his time talking about his previous marriage. Kevin vigorously

regretted getting started with alcohol and blamed his failed marriage on alcohol.

This example highlights the extent to which regret can bind a person to the past. Although there probably is a sizable amount of good information that Kevin could have learned from evaluating his previous behaviors, the influence of regret prevented him from doing so. Kevin's difficulties are likely due to problematic decisions and choices that he made in the past that also hurt people he cared about, and his alcohol abuse may have estranged him from his loved ones. However, regret for these behaviors has made it difficult to shift his focus from the past to the present and then to the future.

Strategies for Managing Regret

Regret can produce an insidious pattern of maladaptive thinking that is difficult for a counselor to challenge. Ingrained patterns of regretful thinking are often supported by highly practiced thoughts that are self-punishing in nature. What makes regret particularly recalcitrant is that most of what is fueling regret are past experiences that cannot be changed. However, there are a few positive aging strategies that can be employed to help a person alter the propensity to engage in regretful thinking. These are highlighted below:

1. Suspend self-judgment: Everyone makes bad decisions.
2. Stop regretful reminiscing by recognizing it and saying: I'm only going to focus on things that I can do something about.
3. Recognize that the world is an imperfect place.

A person who practices regretful thinking will need time and effort to change such patterns. It is easy (and sometimes errantly noble) to feel regretful. The goal of diminishing regret is to understand that at its very core it is a human emotion that reminds a person who has engaged in an offense that the offense was not right. Thus, feeling regret also means that a person has the capacity to self-evaluate his or her own actions. One goal in counseling for regret is to examine specific thinking patterns and the subsequent emotional reactions that occur as a general manifestation of a maladaptive stylistic. It then becomes possible to analyze a situation objectively and to develop alternative ways of reconciling a mistake so as to diminish the negative course of regret.

CONCLUDING COMMENTS

This chapter introduces personality traits that are a stable aspect of a person's intrapsychic world and influence how he or she interacts with the everyday world, including the consequences of personal decisions across the life course. The traits highlighted in this chapter were neuroticism, extraversion, openness to experience, agreeableness, and conscientiousness. For the most part, personality traits are not amenable to change; however, counseling strategies may be effective in altering some of the external manifestations of behavior or cognitive sequelae that result from these traits. For the purpose of developing a general approach to counseling, maladaptive stylistics were identified, including rigidity, negativity, worry, self-absorption, and regret—either as beliefs or assumptions that represent a barrier to positive aging. Each maladaptive stylistic was described as qualitatively distinct; however, the stylistics all reflect an inflated sense of self as deserving exclusive focus from others. Each of these maladaptive characteristics produces a biased form of selective attention on oneself. Counseling strategies were described for assisting older persons who manifest behaviors consistent with rigidity, negativity, worry, self-absorption, and regret.

Chapter 6

PSYCHOTHERAPIES AND
SPECIAL POPULATIONS

TODAY, THE ROLE OF PROFESSIONAL counseling as a way to assist late-life adults in sustaining positive aging is important because mental health concerns extend across the life span; psychological interventions can address normative issues of adaptation in old age in healthy people. Counseling interventions are more accessible and acceptable to the general public (including older adults) than they have been in the past (Hill, Thorn, & Packard, 2000; Cooley, Deitch, et. al., 1998; American Psychological Association, 2004).

MENTAL HEALTH IN OLD AGE:
A LIFE SPAN ISSUE

Mental health issues stretch across the life span and into old age (Areán, 2003). This truism is underscored by prevalence data for two of the most common psychiatric illnesses, namely, depression and anxiety. Clinical depression is a debilitating emotional disorder estimated to afflict between 5 and 10% of the general population (National Institutes of Mental Health, 2001). The symptoms of depression include feelings of hopelessness, loss of pleasure in life, a pervasive sense of guilt and dread, lack of energy, and in more serious cases, the contemplation of suicide (Blazer, 2003). The elderly, as a group, have been characterized as being vulnerable to depression. Epidemiological studies have documented that between 5 and 7% of adults over 65 years of age will experience depression serious enough to require some form of medical intervention (Anthony & Aboraya, 1992), and the suicide risk among older adults is an ongoing public health issue (Turvey et al., 2002).

Research has estimated that some of the highest suicide rates in the general population can be found among elderly people. The Department of Health and Human Services has estimated a suicide rate in the United States of 13.1 per 100,000 persons for adults who were between 65 and 69 years of age (U.S. Department of Health and Human Services, 1999). The reasons enumerated for suicide in late life include a sense of hopelessness, the burden of a chronic physical illness, a sense of isolation or loneliness, combined with substance abuse, and a loss of personal meaning. Suicide is also more likely when older persons are not able to get appropriate mental health care or are unable to access mental health services in a time of need. The high rate of suicide is only one observable phenomenon that underscores the need for effective counseling interventions for persons in late life. Clinical depression and anxiety disorder are risk factors for poor quality of life in old age.

In addition to clinical depression, growing old is associated with a number of risk factors that could trigger depressive symptoms. Living into late life includes a substantial number of challenges, not the least of which are age-related decline in physical health, restrictions in everyday functioning, diminished cognitive functioning, and role loss through retirement, widowhood, and relocation. In addition, aging can be associated with a reduction in available resources including income, social support, and connection to community, all of which could facilitate coping. In the Netherlands the prevalence of depressive symptoms among the elderly has been estimated at almost 13% (Beekman et al., 1995). Rates of depressive symptoms have been found to approach 10% in the United States (Hybels, Blazer, & Pieper, 2001). Depressive symptoms are very amenable to counseling and psychotherapy, and the effectiveness of counseling in particular for alleviating depressive symptoms ranges from good to excellent.

For anxiety, a disorder whose symptoms include subjective distress, nervousness, somatic concerns, racing thoughts, and fear and dread, older adults are particularly vulnerable. Like depression, anxiety can present itself as a formal psychiatric disorder or it can be characterized by the observation of selected symptoms in response to trigger events. As a diagnosable condition, anxiety disorders include panic attack, agoraphobia, and generalized anxiety disorder. These are described below:

Panic attack: Intense fear or discomfort that begins and ends in a short time frame (e.g., 10 minutes). A person may be walking across a street and while doing so experience intense dizziness, trembling, and heart palpitations. This may be followed by fear that one is losing control or dying. Symptoms usually diminish quickly, but can then return at a moment's notice.

Agoraphobia: Fear of going outdoors because one might experience a panic attack or might be harmed in some way. To deal with this, sufferers might become highly ritualistic and rigid. For example, a person might choose to follow a rigidly fixed travel route between home and work with no deviation. Travel outside of this zone could produce severe anxiety.

Generalized Anxiety Disorder (GAD): Fear without an object. For this reason, it is difficult to pinpoint its nature or origin in any given individual. However, it includes chronic, excessive worry, and fear for no real reason. Sufferers tend to worry constantly about everyone and everything in the past and in the future. Examples of worry topics include acceptance from others, family concerns, and poor appraisal of one's personal capabilities. GAD is associated with indecisiveness and a pessimistic view of the future.

Prevalence data suggest that over 8% of the entire adult population may suffer from one of these three forms of anxiety disorder. Among older adults, the Epidemiological Catchment Area Project, one of the most comprehensive surveys of mental health concerns in the United States, estimated that as many as 7% of adults over 65 years of age could be classified with an anxiety disorder. A few studies have suggested that anxiety disorders may be more prevalent in adults over age 65 years than in younger age groups (Goodwin, 2002; Regier et al., 1988). Thus, for those older adults who have symptoms of anxiety, the need for counseling and psychotherapy to help them cope with this emotional disorder has significant public health implications.

It has been estimated that approximately 10% of all older adults experience symptoms of anxiety on a regular basis that would not necessarily meet the diagnostic criteria for a full-blown anxiety disorder as described above (Matt, Dean, Wang & Wood, 1992) This suggests that many older people are likely to encounter a situation that will trigger anxious emotions. In these instances, counseling and psychotherapy might prove helpful in supporting an otherwise healthy individual to deal with a situational anxious state (Wetherell, 1998).

COUNSELING AS A PATHWAY TO POSITIVE AGING

For the larger range of mental health concerns (inclusive of anxiety and depression), the need for counseling and therapy in older adults is strong, even for those issues that would be considered normative in old age including loneliness, caregiving, progressive disability, cognitive decline, and bereavement. It should be noted that these as well as other issues that are part of the aging experience may be associated with a substantial degree of emotional suffering, but they are not necessarily pathological conditions. If one lives long enough, it is inevitable that a loved one will die and the survivor will be confronted with the grief along with the consequences that follow it. Further, the longer one lives the greater the chances of a person becoming a caregiver for an ailing parent, spouse, friend, or sibling. With respect to disability and chronic illness in old age, those people over 85 years of age have a greater than 50% chance of becoming mildly to moderately disabled with respect to everyday activities. These conditions will emerge regardless of whether a person has struggled with anxiety or depression in the past.

Emotional illnesses tend to persist across the life span in that those who have been diagnosed with clinical depression or anxiety disorder in the past are at risk for experiencing those problems again. Counseling may be useful, for example, when a spouse, who has had depression in the past, becomes a caregiver to a partner who unexpectedly experiences cognitive decline due to Alzheimer's disease.

In the 21st century people are living longer, and expect (or hope) that quality of life can be sustained into very old age. Most people not only want to live beyond their average life expectancy, but they also want to have sustained well-being. However, advanced aging is associated with a substantial number of challenges even for someone who has had a relatively problem-free life in youth and adulthood. The thought of experiencing disability and loss, even when it is a normative part of life, can represent, for some, a forbidding psychological challenge. This is true even among the most emotionally hardy persons. It may be that as otherwise healthy adults live into advanced age they may encounter new challenges that can be a source of situational distress. Effective counseling has proven helpful, as a consultation aid, for even the emotionally strong (Hill, Thorn, & Packard, 2000).

Approaches to Counseling Older Adults

The professional field of counseling and psychotherapy has examined an array of therapy strategies. Since the mid 1990s effective approaches have been identified to treat the mental health needs of adults of all ages, including older adults (Duffy, 1999; Gatz et al., 1998; Knight, 1996; Zarit & Knight, 1998). These therapies are known as Empirically Supported Treatments (EST; Deegear & Lawson, 2003). The following list highlights several classes of therapies suggested by Roth and Fonagy (2005) that qualify as EST approaches: psychodynamic therapy; behavioral and cognitive behavioral therapy; family systems therapy; existential therapy.

This list of therapies was also identified by Gatz and colleagues who examined therapy strategies that had support in the empirical literature for specifically addressing older adult needs (Gatz et al. 1998). In their evidenced-based review of treatment approaches, psychodynamic therapy was found to be one of the more efficacious treatments of mood problems in older adults. For anxiety and other similar disorders, behavioral and cognitive behavioral therapies were particularly effective. Life review was recommended as a therapy for issues associated with feeling isolated and alone including dealing with grief and bereavement. Although not specifically highlighted in the Gatz et al. article, family therapy has also been found to be an EST for addressing support issues related to caregiving.

Psychodynamic Therapy

Psychodynamic therapy is based on the concept that personal problems and emotional illness originate in the development of one's personality in early life. Life span oriented models of psychodynamic psychotherapy have argued that because development of the "self" continues across the course of life, a developmental approach to therapy is germane for people in late life. This approach recognizes that there is an unconscious existence where internal or intrapsychic processes actively influence how a person perceives and relates to the world. A critical aspect of this view of the psyche is that people experience conflicts between personal needs or desires and the expectations of society with respect to their behavior. The human psyche, in this regard, must balance these conflicts through conscious reconciliation processes that are sensitive to the person's interpersonal world.

This approach acknowledges that development of personality continues across the life span. It embodies models of life span maturation, such as those espoused by Erikson (1963; Erikson, Erikson, & Kivnick 1986) and Jung (1933), both of whom believed that the resolution of internal needs in relation to the external world is an essential component to optimal adaptation. The goal of therapy is to resolve difficulties associated with life stages, and in the process, cultivate maturational characteristics (e.g., hope). Jung also viewed adult development with respect to stages or phases across the life span, seeing life as consisting of three phases: youth, middle age, and old age. With respect to the latter two phases, Jung saw middle age as a period of questioning long-held convictions, and old age as a period of increased introspection and self-evaluation. These processes are precisely those needed in order for a psychodynamic approach to counseling to be effective.

The process of counseling and psychotherapy, from a psychodynamic perspective, focuses on conscious understanding of verbal descriptions of internal states of conflict and how these are manifested in a person's relationships with others or how they emerge in a self-appraisal of personal motivations. The specific approach of psychodynamic therapy involves helping the individual alter his or her psychological state through developing alternative patterns of relating to problems rather than repeating strategies that were developed by the individual as a result of past intra- or interpersonal conflicts. For interpersonal issues, the tensions between dependence and independence are very important. The specific approach to therapy involves the client finding new understanding about past losses and conflicts, especially as these are related to separation and individuation. The client's new understandings, then, emerge as part of the therapeutic relationship that is constructed, with assistance from the therapist, to be a context within which the client can work through past conflicts that have led the client (or made him or her vulnerable) to engage in maladaptive ways of thinking and coping.

A client who, for example, was heavily ridiculed as a child by his father, may have, in the process of early development, arrived at a view of the world that dictates denying the existence of internal needs as a way to deal with those very needs. Such a rigid and self-effacing approach to negotiating an internal conflict could lead to a profound source of anxiety when an intrapersonal desire or urge, such as a sexual feeling toward another person, becomes conscious. In this instance, the psychodynamic therapist would encourage the client to explore the origin of his or her feelings with the hope of developing insight into the issue or problem. It then becomes possible to guide the client in finding new ways of dealing with old patterns of coping.

Considerable research has emerged regarding the use of psychodynamic therapy in the treatment of older adults who experience emotional illnesses such as depression (Morgan & Goldstein, 2003), as well as for issues that are often part of the older adult life experience such as caregiving (Gallagher-Thompson & Steffen, 1994). A vignette illustrating the application of psychodynamic therapy follows:

> Mary was a 75-year-old mother of three and grandmother of seven. She and her husband, Herb, were happily married for over 50 years, and although they had marital problems from

time to time, their relationship improved as they grew into old age. Mary's youngest son Danny, 38, had an alcohol problem for most of his life. He had been hospitalized twice and struggled with bouts of depression. Shortly before Danny's birthday he had a severe argument with Mary. This argument revolved around the point that Mary felt Danny was the only one of her three children who had experienced a ruined life. Danny left their home after the argument and ceased contact with his parents. The week after the argument he was driving to a party while under the influence of alcohol and hit a tree. The impact killed him and two of his friends. This traumatic event left Mary wondering if she had been more understanding of Danny and his problems he might not have been killed in this way. Mary has had difficulty sleeping and has been disturbed by dreams of Danny scolding her. Mary felt that Danny's death was partly her responsibility and that if she had been a better mother to him he might not have engaged in alcohol abuse. Mary felt guilty most of the time, had not been eating well, felt hopeless, and was unable to get any pleasure out of life. Her life seemed frozen at the point of this incident. She wondered if she could keep on living knowing that Danny's death may have been, in some way, related to her harshness.

Mary was encouraged by her oldest brother to seek professional counseling. She retained a psychologist who, in the first session, took a detailed history of her life, including her relationship with Danny. They worked together to identify Mary's feelings of guilt about Danny. A central aspect of therapy was to identify the points of conflict between Danny and his mother. This process identified a dynamic between Mary and her son whereby she had been emotionally unwilling to let Danny develop his independence. This may have been due to the fact that he was the youngest child. Further exploration revealed, however, that Mary had engaged in this same dependency dynamic with all of her children. Danny, it seemed, had more difficulty than the others in individuating from her. This became worse when Danny was not able to change his alcohol abuse patterns and could not independently support himself. The therapist and Mary explored the nature of Danny's addiction and what it meant with respect to his dependency needs.

Mary looked forward to the appointments with the therapist and felt that she was understood. Most of the time she left a session with some concrete ideas for addressing her problem. Slowly, through the course of therapy, Mary began to let go of her need to be responsible for Danny's tragedy and, as she did so, she was able to be freer with her other children. As her self-evaluation changed, her behaviors toward others improved. Over time, she was also able to put Danny into the background of her mind so that she could get on with life. In a sense, she let Danny go.

At the end of therapy, Mary felt more worthwhile and again began to enjoy living. It was difficult for Mary to leave therapy, but the counselor encouraged her to follow through and to find new sources of meaning outside therapy that she could use to address future problems and issues.

This case highlights the essential steps of psychodynamic therapy. These are: (1) Take a relevant history of the client with respect to the problem or issue. (2) Develop a meaningful relationship with the client. (3) Define the presenting problem(s). (4) Actively convey a sense of optimism to the client. (5) Proceed to address the presenting problem. (6) Focus primarily on the present. (7) Place emphasis on deepening the therapist–client relationship. (8) Address issues of loss and abandonment. (9) Support the patient's ego strength. (10) Strengthen the client's sense of self as worthwhile (Knight, 1996 & Garmer, 2002).

Psychodynamic therapy is a powerful technique, particularly for issues that impact the parent–child relationship, the most salient of which is the dependent–independent dynamic as described in Mary's case. However, psychodynamic therapy is not restricted to this issue and can be employed for a range of problems. It is an excellent tool for the treatment of clinical depression. A stereotypical assumption is that this form of therapy requires many sessions and years of treatment to achieve gains. The empirical literature does not support this notion. In fact, the modal approach for psychodynamic therapy requires less than 12 weeks of treatment (Crits-Christoph & Barber, 1991).

Behavioral and Cognitive Behavioral Therapy

Behavioral and cognitive behavioral therapy (CBT) have emerged from a number of theoretical sources, including behaviorism and cognitive psychology. The underlying assumption is that behavior can influence one's emotional state, and how one thinks can have emotional consequences. Behavioral therapy assumes that when a patient changes his or her behavior in a positive direction, discomfort/distress will diminish. Therapy involves both recognizing the emotional consequences of one's behavior and learning to practice new behaviors that are incompatible with negative emotional consequences.

CBT takes this notion a bit further and adds thought processes to the therapeutic mix. Specifically, how one thinks and behaves influences how one feels. The goal of CBT is to alter what have formerly been maladaptive patterns of behaving, thinking, or believing (e.g., irrational beliefs) in order to restore one's sense of emotional well-being or reduce psychological symptoms. The variations in these therapies are due, in part, to the wide range of intervention techniques that can be employed under the umbrella of the CBT approach. These techniques increase the performance of behaviors that are associated with positive affect and include, self-monitoring of maladaptive thoughts, challenging erroneous and competing assumptions ("Being old is being ugly," or "I must be told that I am beautiful in order to feel good about myself"), relaxation training through controlled breathing exercises, and setting up rewards for behavior that promote well-being.

Although the list of specific CBT techniques is long, a theme that ties them together involves altering the external environment or how one thinks about the environment, in order to facilitate adaptation or positive aging. Unlike the psychodynamic model described earlier, this approach deemphasizes the inherent and developmental nature of one's intrapersonal world. The focus is on what can be done to improve a person's current state of functioning in the world. With respect to behavioral and CBT as ESTs specific to older adults, considerable evidence indicates that these approaches can be effective in dealing with a wide variety of mental health issues (Coon et al., 1999; Hyer, Kramer, & Schule, 2004; Scholey & Woods, 2003; Stanley & Novy, 2000).

In one study (Wetherell, Gatz, & Craske, 2003) that involved a collection of behavioral and cognitive behavioral procedures that have been validated in the professional literature, including relaxation training (Scogin, Rickard, Keith, Wilson, McElreath, 1992), cognitive restructuring, and worry exposure, an effort was made to test whether such treatments could reduce symptoms of anxiety in 75 older individuals who were 55 years of age and over and who carried diagnoses of generalized anxiety disorder. Treatment involved *relaxation training* by systematically focusing on bodily sensations and controlled breathing; *cognitive restructuring* (Hyer et al., 2004) that involved challenging the client's thought distortions (e.g., "I must be liked by everyone in order to be happy") with more adaptive ways of thinking (e.g., "It would be nice to be liked by everybody, but my happiness does not depend on others opinions about me"); and *worry exposure* (Borkovec, Shadick, & Hopkins, 1991), which involved practicing resolving worry experiences where the experiences were graded with respect to their traumatic impact (e.g., low—you might have offended the driver who just passed you on the road; high—you might have offended your employer and put your job in jeopardy). The CBT therapy manual that was used in this study was specific to older adults and adapted from a more general training manual (Craske, Barlow, & O'Leary, 1992). The manual taught the clients about anxiety, how to monitor and control it, and how to reduce it through the techniques noted above. An important aspect of this study (Wetherell et al., 2003) was that the treatment condition group was contrasted to both a wait-list control group, and, a focused discussion group. In the focused discussion group, participants were asked to simply discuss the topic of anxiety. At a six-month follow-up, over half of those in the CBT group reported meaningful improvement with respect to reducing their anxiety symptoms, and 29% reported a marked reduction in anxiety. There was no evidence of change in anxiety symptoms in the two control conditions.

This study is important for several reasons. First, the approach is very concrete and time limited. Thus, it could be adapted to address a number of problems. Second, it was conducted with older adults as clients, which provides evidence that older adults can benefit from treatment. Third, therapists followed a manual, which reduces the likelihood that treatment group participants got better because of therapist charisma. The use of manuals also demonstrates that it is possible for professionals to learn effective skills for treating older clients with emotional issues.

In a related study (Stanley et al., 2003) CBT was examined in contrast to a control group that involved regular contact with clients, but no active intervention. Participants in this study were 85 older adults (60 years and older) who were diagnosed with generalized anxiety disorder (GAD). Recall that GAD consists of excessive worry, vague symptoms of discomfort or fear that is difficult to pinpoint, and somatic concerns. Participants were randomly assigned to one of two groups. In the treatment group, participants engaged in education and awareness training about the nature of their anxiety and were taught progressive muscle relaxation. Cognitive training, which represented the core approach to treatment, consisted of teaching these participants to challenge many of their misconceptions that were at the root of their anxiety, including the propensity for worrying excessively. An example of such misconceptions involved irrational thinking errors such as "My world is falling apart" or "Something is wrong with me." The therapist engaged the clients to change these thoughts in ways that would lower anxiety, for example, "Something in my life is not right, but I can work on this issue until I feel better about it."

An innovative aspect of the CBT treatment in this study involved participants creating a 10-item hierarchy of anxiety-producing stimuli or situations. The therapist then helped the clients confront and work through each of these situations (in the presence of deep muscle relaxation). One goal of this process was to help the client feel better about encountering such situations in real life. In some instances, in order to help the treatment generalize beyond the therapy context, participants were instructed to confront the real-life situation during the course of therapy. This form of therapy was highly effective in helping the treatment participants reduce their level of anxiety symptoms. In the treatment group, 45% of the participants reported a reduction in their symptoms versus only 8% in the minimal contact/education control group. Of most importance here, however, was the finding that participants in the treatment group reported substantial reductions in their anxiety symptoms one year after the treatment was over.

Taken together, these two studies (Stanley et al., 2003; Wetherell et al., 2003) underscore the effectiveness of cognitive behavioral training for older adults. Cognitive behavioral therapy is an appealing treatment alternative because it is very straightforward, involves direct education about the client's symptoms and concerns, engages the client in a meaningful way to reduce symptoms, and does not require a large number of sessions in order for clients to experience an appreciable reduction in their symptoms. Thus, it may represent the therapy of choice when dealing with issues related to depression or anxiety.

The case study below highlights the process and structure of a typical case of an older adult with anxious symptoms who benefited from CBT. Embedded in this case are the essential components of the treatment that are summarized in the section that follows:

> Karen was 63 years old and single. She worked as a teacher in a local high school. Karen's primary complaint was that she was experiencing bouts of anxiety without any apparent source. She said, "During the day I have these persistent feelings that I am falling apart and losing my mind." In a recent instance during a class that she was teaching she had the profound feeling that she was losing control of herself and that she needed to leave the room. It was at this point that she became unable to speak without great effort, so she ended the class abruptly. She reported that these kinds of events were happening more often and other teachers and the principal began noticing.

CBT began with the therapist assisting Karen in identifying several thinking errors that she engaged in just prior to these anxious feelings. Two thoughts that frequently occurred were: (1) "If I make a mistake the students will laugh at me"; and (2) "I must get this lecture perfect or I am not a worthwhile instructor and I should retire and let someone younger and better take my place." With respect to the first thought, Karen described an event where she had made an error in working out a math problem and the student who corrected her made a derogatory remark during the class. Although she dismissed this student from class, his remark continued to bother her.

The therapist educated Karen about the relationship between assumptions that people make about themselves and others and how those assumptions can get distorted and then ultimately affect one's sense of well-being. The therapist suggested that Karen challenge this thinking. It was decided that she would track how often she was laughed at in class. She discovered, over time, that this event rarely occurred, and when it did, it was unrelated to her actual performance. The therapist then helped Karen challenge her maladaptive thought pattern by reframing it as follows: "It would be nice if people would not laugh at me if I make a mistake, but that doesn't mean that I am a failure." Karen was asked to practice this alternative thought. As Karen began to successfully challenge her maladaptive thought patterns, her perception of herself and her capabilities improved. Interestingly, on one occasion, a group of students did laugh at her for putting the wrong homework on the board. Prior to therapy, this might have upset her to the point that she would miss work the next day. However, in this instance, she simply erased the error, put the correct homework up, and moved on without incident or worry. Her comment to the therapist was, "When you are a teacher, showing how to recover from mistakes is part of being a good role model to students."

This case example highlights the essential steps of CBT, which are outlined below. It is important to note that the critical element of this kind of therapy is learning how to challenge errant thought patterns when these are unrealistic and maladaptive. Following this, the therapist helps the client replace those thoughts with thinking that is more realistic and that the client can act on in order to reduce his or her anxious or depressive symptoms.

- Define the presenting problem(s).
- Identify maladaptive thought patterns.
- Take a strategic history of the client to better understand the origins of the maladaptive thoughts.
- Teach a form of relaxation technique and encourage the client to practice these skills during therapy and at home.
- Teach the client how to challenge maladaptive thoughts.
- During therapy, help the client practice challenging maladaptive thoughts.
- Give the client homework, so he or she can practice challenging maladaptive thoughts in the real world (the patient keeps a diary or record of these efforts).

- Support the client's learning.
- Strengthen the client's sense of control over thoughts and feelings.

CBT is, perhaps, the most common mode of therapy that is employed in working with older adults, and there is a wealth of literature supporting this therapy (Gorenstein, Papp, & Kleber, 1996; Hyer et al., 2004; Qualls, 2004; Stanley & Novy, 2000; Wetherell, 1998). One of the appealing aspects of CBT is its straightforward technique. Strategies such as relaxation training, coping skills training, and self-management have become an integral part of a variety of health-care contexts for treating a range of conditions from headaches to cigarette smoking. CBT doesn't require an extensive clinical history, nor does it make assumptions about how past dynamics are influencing a current situation. For some people, the kind of focus found in CBT is what they need in order to make progress on an issue or problem. [An excellent general reference for CBT techniques is Dobson, 2000.]

Family Systems Therapy

A large number of issues that face older adults involve interpersonal relationships within families. Noteworthy among these is caregiving, grief or bereavement, retirement, and relationship issues that emerge when children leave the home. Caregiving represents one of the more significant family-associated challenges in old age. It has been estimated that as many as one out of four households (or 22.4 million families) is involved in caring for an older loved one who has some form of age-related disability (AARP, 2001). It is not surprising, then, that caregiving not only is a significant personal and societal concern but is associated with a high degree of individual and family burdens including anxiety, distress, and depression. For this reason, there is a pressing need for effective therapies that can assist families in coping with the psychological consequences of caregiving. The individual approaches to therapy summarized above—psychodynamic therapy and cognitive behavioral therapy—can be helpful, but often the primary issue is not just individual, but involves the entire family system.

133

With this in mind, it should be noted that although therapies that focus on family interaction patterns did not develop with the older adult in mind and have a more diffuse history than other therapeutic paradigms such as psychodynamic and behavioral approaches, they are well suited to dealing with a class of issues that represent one of the more pressing public health needs among older Americans; that is, caregiving (Florsheim & Herr, 1990).

With respect to the treatment of older adults who are caregivers, it is important to identify strategies or techniques that have received empirical support in the literature for producing positive outcomes (Mitrani & Czaja, 2000). Several of the prominent strategies are: (1) communication skills training; (2) group interaction management; and (3) relationship enhancement.

Communication skills training involves the systematic assessment and management of messages (verbal and nonverbal) to maximize coping. Herr and Weakland (1979) identified three levels of communication in this regard. The first level involves content or the actual meaning of spoken communication (e.g., "My partner is not a bother to me"). The second level involves the emotional meaning of the message (e.g., a sarcastic vs. a sincere tone). The third level is the nonverbal language of the individual (e.g., sitting with legs crossed and arms folded). The goal of communications skills training is to help family members send messages that are consistent across these three levels of communication. A mixed message is delivered when a client verbally indicates that his spouse does not bother him, while his tone and nonverbal language indicates that there is something wrong in the relationship.

Group interaction management is employed to minimize the frequency with which a mixed message is sent. This is a particularly important therapeutic technique when age-related transitions alter the stable nature of a family dynamic such as when the husband or wife leaves the workforce through retirement. A change in lifestyle behaviors may require substantial adjustments in how individual family members relate to (or work around) one another. If mixed messages across these levels of communication become frequent and common, families will have difficulty adapting to changed lifestyle patterns (e.g., "I used to be able to tolerate his sarcasm about me when I knew he would be at work, but now that he is retired I can't escape from him").

There is some evidence that family-based therapies that proactively engage group interaction management and support of family members who are caring for an elderly loved one, particularly how they approach one another in alleviating sources of distress, can be helpful for reducing caregiver burdens (Benbow & Mariott, 1997; Zarit & Knight, 1996). The essential concept is that through group interaction management the therapist encourages family members to engage in active discussion and interaction in topics that are causing psychological stress. This, then, provides opportunities for family members to show direct support for one another and to problem solve ways in which the family might communicate more clearly about a shared psychological burden. This idea has been suggested by a number of prominent geropsychologists including Steven Zarit and colleagues (Zarit, Anthony, & Boutselis 1987) as an effective strategy for dealing with caregiver burden. These ideas have been integrated in several large-scale interventions such as the Resources for Enhancing Alzheimer's Caregiver Health (REACH; Wisniewski et al., 2003) that focus on the family unit as the vehicle for facilitating the coping of individuals who are experiencing emotional distress due to caregiving (Czaja, Schulz, Chin Lee, & Belle, 2003).

The third strategy, *relationship enhancement,* can also be found as a core element in couples counseling for marital satisfaction. One aspect of relationship enhancement is assisting those in the relationship to be more sensitive and supportive of age-related changes from the "other" person's perspective. Rosowsky (1999) described several relationship enhancement techniques that involve helping individuals within the family relationship (or marriage) understand that each member of the unit may be at differing stages of development (or maturation) and for this reason may view a problem and its apparent solution from a very different perspective. Relationship enhancement involves encouraging open collaboration, affirmation of one another, as well as respecting each member of the relationship. It is a technique that can be a profound source of growth as well as healing, particularly when one of the members of the relationship suffers from an emotional health problem (Benbow & Mariott, 1997).

The case study below highlights a situation that could benefit from a family systems approach to therapy. Although one spouse was in the early stage of Alzheimer's disease, there were still benefits from intervening systemically. This case also highlights the eclectic nature of the treatment components that make up family therapy:

Mary and James had been happily married for 53 years. James had been an aircraft mechanic for most of his life and Mary had her own sewing business that she ran out of their home. Mary and James had three sons, all married (although two of her sons had divorced and remarried). None of their sons had children from any relationship, so Mary was not a grandmother, and she highlighted this as one of her biggest disappointments in life. Recently, James began to notice that Mary was experiencing some memory problems. These problems started as signs of forgetfulness and apparent inattention; however, they got progressively worse as Mary had more and more trouble saying words, remembering where she was (even when at home) and got lost in her own neighborhood and forgot the names of familiar people in her world, including her sons' spouses. In fact, one of the more embarrassing issues in this regard was Mary's propensity to mention the sons' exspouses when the sons came to visit. As Mary's problems became worse, Joe was not well equipped to deal with these issues psychologically, so he resorted to drinking alcohol, which also impaired his functioning. The couple had never been in mental health counseling before; however, recently, when Mary was having problems, Joe attempted to drive her to a son's house. Joe had been drinking and was stopped by the police and issued a DUI citation. He was so intoxicated at the time, that the police held him overnight and released Mary into the custody of her son. The couple was subsequently court-ordered to receive counseling. Part of the counseling involved family therapy.

During the course of therapy, the therapist encouraged Joe and Mary's sons to attend sessions and they did this without hesitation.

One aspect of the counseling was to identify patterns in the family that created barriers between the couple and their sons' relationship with them. One of the biggest barriers was Mary's insistence on bringing up the marital history of each son. Because Mary was unable to inhibit this, a strategy was created whereby when Mary began to talk in this way, she was asked to leave the room where she could be distracted by watching a VCR tape of her favorite television show. Because her memory was short, this was very effective in alleviating some of the bad feelings that often ensued when Mary was not stopped. Additionally, the sons were able to bring current spouses to several of the sessions, so that the spouses could learn more about the context around Mary's social misbehavior. Slowly, and over a long period of time, the family began to accept this aspect of Mary's impairment and it became less of a problem. The solution to this issue was also helpful for Joe as well, and he was able to talk about trigger situations that put him at risk for drinking alcohol. The family was able to discuss Joe's drinking problem as a group, including one of Joe's sons who also had a history of alcohol problems. Together, the family was able to develop several general strategies to assist Joe in controlling his drinking behavior.

This case highlights the essential steps of family systems therapy. These steps are outlined below:

- Take a relevant history of each person in the family system.
- Define the presenting problem(s) from a systems perspective.
- Help the family set achievable therapy goals to address the problem.
- Maintain the focus on the problem and not on any specific individual.
- Encourage an open process welcoming different viewpoints.
- Focus on how relationships can adapt to address issues.
- Facilitate the general system.
- Avoid systemic bias and identify it when it appears.
- Interpret meaning from group discussions.
- Keep a focus on the problem and its resolution.

Family systems therapy is an essential tool for the practitioner who desires to provide mental health services to older adults who are caregivers. Many problems encountered in old age are from within the context of a family system. It is this system that can both facilitate and undercut a person's efforts to change or adapt. Further, for certain kinds of issues such as marital concerns, caregiving, parent and adult child issues, family systems therapy may be the only way to approach the problem. Individual therapy for a marital concern might make sense for a small number of issues, but it is very difficult to address issues in a long-term marital relationship without having both partners present. The effectiveness of family systems therapy is generally good for issues noted above as they emerge over the life span. There are a number of good references that can be consulted when using family systems therapy with older adults (Florsheim & Herr, 1990; Herr & Weakland, 1979; Mitrani & Czaja, 2000; Mittelman, Epstein, & Pierzchala, 2002; Rosowsky, E., 1999).

Existential Therapy

Existential therapy is an approach to counseling that, in a conceptual sense, is ideally suited to the older client because it focuses on the person's sense of authenticity and meaning. The existential approach is less technique (or strategy) driven than the therapies described previously; instead, it focuses on the cultivation of meaning and finding personal growth and development by engaging in self-evaluation and self-understanding as these relate to a specific issue or challenge. Emphasis in existential therapy is placed on the individual as the agent of change; however, change is the result of an ongoing effort that the individual exerts on developing his or her personal sources of meaning and self-awareness. Although the roots of existential therapy come from the writings of well-known thinkers, philosophers, and scholars such as Kierkegaard and Nietzsche, existential psychotherapists such as Rollo May, and others have provided a framework for using such philosophical ideas to address a wide range of emotional issues including anxiety, loneliness, grief, and depression (Frankl, 1985; Kierkegaard, 1970; May, 1983; Nietzsche, 1958; van Deurzen, 2002; Yalom, 1980). In his book, *Psychology and the Human Dilemma* (1967), May described the experience of anxiety in this way:

We have noted some problems which arise from the loss of individual significance. This loss forces us all to confront the struggle to find and preserve personal identity. The pain of which I speak—and indeed the common denominator as we all experience it in such dilemmas—is anxiety. Neurotic anxiety is destructive. It consists of shrinking of consciousness, the blocking off of awareness; and when it is prolonged it leads to a feeling of depersonalization and apathy. (pp 40–41)

Lantz and Raiz (2004) reported results of an informal study that utilized an existential approach in marital therapy with a group of 26 couples (65 years and older). In this study, existential therapy was operationalized as four basic intervention strategies; holding, telling, mastering, and honoring. *Holding* was defined as the relational context that the therapist creates with the client. In this instance, the goal of therapy is to engage a relationship where empathy and mutual understanding are engendered. This kind of interpersonal environment opens the door to deeper exploration of the client's presenting concerns. *Telling* involves client self-disclosure about the nature and psychological experience of the client's presenting concerns. This includes expression of existential pain. The process of disclosure also allows the person, with therapist guidance, to reframe their issue or concern so that it is more manageable and modifiable with effort. *Mastery* involves the client acting on his or her own emotional pain with the goal of resolving or accepting it. Successfully reducing existential pain may involve efforts on the client's part to engage psychological strategies including reframing, thoughtful reflection, or even objectively changing the client's interpersonal world (moving away from one's adult children). The final step, *honoring*, is when healing occurs. This involves learning to acknowledge the fact that intrapersonal pain is a necessary and unavoidable part of human existence and that finding meaning in one's own suffering can represent a source of maturation and growth even in old age. To some extent this four-component model is consistent with many of the more contemporary approaches to existential therapy for adults without respect to age (Wong, 2004).

In their study, Lantz and Raiz (2004) treated each couple for an average of 18 sessions across a four- to six-month time interval.

Several paper-and-pencil measures were administered to the couples at intake, termination, and after six months. These instruments included The Purpose in Life Test (Crumbaugh & Maholick, 1964) as well as the Marital Relationship Perceptions Test (Lantz, 1975). The couples showed positive change on both of these instruments from intake to termination and even after six months. Because there was no control group, it was not possible to reliably rule out spontaneous improvement in these older couples with time; however, Lantz and Raiz (2004) recorded the verbal reports from these older couples that were affirming of therapy as enhancing their sense of meaning and understanding of themselves in the world, as well as improving their marital problems.

For the counselor who desires to use existential therapy with older clients, studies like the one described above suggest that this approach has promise for ameliorating psychological problems that are associated with relationships as well as individual personal meaning. Specific issues that are amenable to this kind of approach include marital dissatisfaction, relationship issues with adult children, caregiver concerns, loneliness, anxiety, and depression. Although the stereotype that existential therapy is too abstract to use with older persons is very persistent, gerontology counselors who use the existential approach argue that it is particularly well suited for older adults because the approach focuses on real people facing realistic human problems that if not resolved, have predictable life-span consequences. Langle (2004) described existential psychotherapy as: "a psychotherapeutic method to help people to come to live with inner consent to their own actions" (p. 100). In this regard, existential therapy may be the treatment of choice when dealing with an older person who has a clear sense of values and has developed a sense of meaning through which adaptation occurs.

Life Review Therapy

Specific to older adults, a variant of the existential approach as articulated by Robert Butler is life review therapy (Butler, 1974). A life review, also called reminiscence therapy (Butler, 1963; Rando, 2000), is a therapeutic approach that acknowledges the importance of meaning as a source of positive aging. Life review therapy involves the active process of recollecting life events in such a way as to gain better perspective over one's present situation. In this case, an issue may be contemplating the end of one's own life in very advanced age (provided the intellect is intact) or following the death of a loved one, such as a spouse. In many ways, life review is not only consistent with continuity theory, and the view that change and adaptation are normal developmental processes, but it also emphasizes the importance of increasing awareness of one's mortality.

The process of life review begins with the therapist guiding the older client through a recollection of past experiences to help the person cope with a current life challenge or problem. The concept is that the past can help the older adult find new meaning to replace a present loss. Butler described the goal of life review therapy as assisting a person in maintaining a consistent sense of self in the face of age-related change (Molinari, 1999).

Life review therapy in its various forms has been found to be effective in helping older adults cope with depression, particularly when it is caused by a current life situation such as the loss of a loved one or the emergence of age-related disability in contexts including nursing homes (Rattenberg & Stones, 1989). Life review is as effective as CBT for the treatment of depression, with the advantage that life review therapy is much more consistent with how an older adult might naturally cope with an emotional health issue. In many ways, life review embodies the notion of positive aging in that it is an approach that affirms an individual's uniqueness and personal capabilities to meet and overcome challenges. By applying past successes (and failures) to cope with a psychological challenge, the individual can capitalize on the unique coping characteristics that are the most salient for any given individual (Butler, 1974).

The example below demonstrates the principles of life review therapy and emphasizes the essential components of continuity theory and how these work through Life Review Therapy to help an older adult negotiate age-related disability and impending death in old age.

Steve, a financially successful real estate developer, was recently diagnosed with supranuclear palsy, a debilitating age-related disease that profoundly impairs motor function. Initially, Steve ignored this diagnosis, a coping strategy that he had developed over the years for dealing with unwanted issues in his life. Steve was a devout Catholic for most of his life and he had lived for many years in an unhappy marriage that ended after 30 years in a bitter divorce. This union had produced 10 children and there were multiple issues that the children were involved in regarding the divorce process. After Steve's divorce, he married a Jewish woman who was 20 years his junior. This had estranged him from his Catholic roots and had further strained his relationship with several of his children, who viewed him as a "cradle robber."

In seeking professional help, Steve met with a geriatric health care practitioner for several sessions. In the first three sessions, the counselor encouraged Steve to retell his family history. Through this process Steve was able to talk about the difficulty of his first marriage, the reasons he chose to leave the marriage, and the work he had done to ensure that his ex-spouse was financially cared for even though he felt that she had not appreciated his generosity in this regard. He also was able to talk about the factors that motivated his decision to remarry outside the Catholic faith.

The counselor carefully assisted Steve in constructing a new image for himself, one that involved his ability to deal with adversity, his coping strategies, and how he wanted to be viewed after his death. Although Steve was not able to reconcile the anguish that he believed he had caused his ex-spouse and several of his children, the counselor helped Steve to focus on the variety of responses that his children had expressed about his personal and family decisions. Through this process of life review, Steve was able to release some of the animosity he held toward his ex-wife and the feelings of regret he had with respect to some of his children. He was also able to acknowledge that as his symptoms became worse, his current wife and several of his children would be there for him and that, in this way, his legacy as a "provider" to his children would not be lost when he eventually died.

The therapist engaged Steve in a meaningful review of his past as a way to identify themes that could be used to help him find a larger sense of meaning and purpose in his life. Steve's participation in this process required him to let go of his compartmentalization strategy in order to realistically describe himself and his motives. It was at that point that the therapist encouraged Steve to construct a broader, more meaningful sense of himself from a life span perspective. As Steve internalized this perspective he found ways to reconcile himself with parts of his life that, before the intervention, seemed inconsistent. Life review therapy was a vehicle that helped Steve develop a more realistic appraisal of himself and his life choices from a broader set of parameters acknowledging that life (and living life) can be disappointing and hard, but that it is also possible to find peace of mind and contentment if one can focus on the larger life span themes.

Several distinguishing features of life review therapy can be gleaned from this case study. Initially, Steve was unable to accept his impending decline and death and this prevented him from acknowledging his own mortality and dealing with it from a more mature perspective. As therapy progressed, Steve was able to realize that his physical decline and death were unavoidable, which freed him to fully explore his life and its meaning.

Through strategic reminiscence, Steve was also able to identify and acknowledge his need to compartmentalize his issues. And as he slowly became able to reexamine his life from a more holistic and integrated perspective, his mood improved. Although life review revealed both the good and bad that had resulted from decisions he had made earlier in his life, he was able to develop a more realistic appraisal of how his motives had changed from one of self-interest to a focus on others who were important to him, including his children and his current spouse. As he did this he was able to cultivate a sense of gratitude for them. In the end, Steve's self-view gradually shifted from a deprived, lonely invalid who feared dying, to someone who had made an effort to cope with living in his own way in an imperfect world. As he engaged this changed self-image his desire to reconnect with his family and loved ones increased.

The essential steps of life review therapy include: The acknowledgment that life is temporary; strategic reminiscences of the meaningful past; positive reframing of unresolved conflicts from a life span perspective; integrating elements of the past into a current sense of self (Watt & Cappeliez, 1995; Watt & Wong, 1991). Life review therapy is only one form of existential therapy; however, it is

143

described here because unlike psychodynamic, CBT, and family systems therapy, it was pioneered with the older client in mind (Butler, 1963, 1974). Data also supports this approach as particularly meaningful for older adults who are dealing with end-of-life issues (Molinari & Reichlin, 1985). Special themes may arise during life review therapy including helping older clients resolve issues of meaning in their individual lives through values clarification, addressing spiritual issues associated with the dying process, and assisting the client in creating meaning and a legacy. It is important that practitioners who work with older adults develop skills in this therapy approach.

Group Counseling

Older adults reside in a variety of contexts beyond the home, including residential care facilities, board and care homes, and hospitals (Hill, Thorn, Bowling, & Morrison, 2002). Those who live at home could be homebound and unable to travel to a therapist's office. Further, issues facing older adults, such as caregiving, may benefit from therapy that incorporates multiple mechanisms for support beyond the therapist.

Group counseling is an alternative mode of therapy that could address some of these issues. In many ways, it is more efficient than individual therapy because multiple persons can be treated in a single session. Further, there are many positive consequences from group therapy, especially when it is managed by a skilled leader. Of particular benefit is the support and encouragement a person can receive from other group members, as well as the opportunity to hear about how others are struggling with a common problem. For older adults, several examples of traditional contexts where group therapy may be preferred over individual therapy are listed below.

- Traditional Group Counseling Approaches
    Support
            Caregiver support groups
            Widow support groups
    Skills
            Social skills groups
            Activity groups (learning a new skill)

Behavior change
  Exercise groups
  Weight loss groups
  Smoking cessation groups
  Alcohol and narcotics abstinence groups (AA, NA)
Mental health treatment
  Depression
  Anxiety
• Innovative Group Counseling Approaches
Relationship enhancement
  Friendship groups
  Marital/family enhancement groups
Study
  Current events discussion groups
  Book groups
Topical
  Volunteering or service-learning groups
  Charity donation group
  Community-service group

Traditional group contexts revolve around the provision of support, as is highlighted in caregiver and widow support groups (Stewart, Craig, MacPherson, & Alexander, 2001). The goal of support groups is to give people who are struggling with a common issue the benefit of interacting with others who are dealing with similar issues. These kinds of groups can be open ended to encourage free discussion or they can have an educational theme that is germane to a specific issue. A topic for a caregiver support group might be, "How to access respite services." In this case, the group may share ideas about accessing respite services or there could be an organized curriculum that includes a featured speaker who is an expert in the area.

Support groups are ubiquitous and can be found in many community, medical, and professional contexts. Attendance at these groups is often free because of sponsorship by organizations such as the National Alzheimer's Association. Groups can also be sponsored by local businesses, as is often the case for widow support groups that may be supported by local funeral homes. In many instances, attendance does not have a set time limit. This allows for significant social support to develop. It has been estimated that between 10 and 15% of all caregivers will attend an organized caregiver support group. Assuming that the number of caregivers in the United States is 65 million (or one third of the adult population) this would mean that between 6 and 7 million people seek help through caregiver support groups annually (AARP, 2001)

Skills groups, behavior change groups, and mental health treatment groups are less prevalent than support groups, given that skill training involves a much more thematic approach and the target population is smaller than is typical for support groups. The goal of thematic groups is defined by the topic or activity from which the group was constructed. If an older adult is isolated, a social skills group might be a way to learn strategies for building a social network. Whereas support groups can often be informally led, thematic groups are led by a skilled leader or an expert in the area. This is particularly the case when the expectation is that the group will address a mental health issue such as depression. For mental health treatment, there is an extensive literature that argues for the beneficial effects of group psychotherapy for adults who range in age across the life span (Burlingame, Fuhriman, & Mosier, 2003; Burlingame, MacKenzie, & Strauss, 2004; Molinari, 1999).

The effectiveness of group treatment can be optimized in three ways: (1) proper structuring of the composition of the group with respect to the type of problem and severity of the issue. In this regard, the more homogeneous group membership has a better outcome; (2) use of a highly skilled leader who has expertise with respect to the thematic issue or problem, as well as experience in leading groups on this topic; (3) designing a format that incorporates active treatment activities and that provides an opportunity for participants to interact in a meaningful way. This latter guideline is especially important for behavior change groups, which have been found to be more effective when the curriculum is concrete and well organized.

There are several recent innovations in group therapy that take advantage of social dynamics to promote positive aging. Study groups are a format for learning new information about a topic or event with the goal that the group format will promote discussion and interaction among participants. A fascinating example of this is the study circle concept, which has been used extensively in Sweden as an informal way to promoting adult continuing education. These are state sponsored and financially supported groups composed of three or more adults that address topics of common interest to the participants. In the study circle, participants engage in an exchange of ideas, critical thinking, and the application of knowledge. It is hoped that they learn to speak and listen in the group and develop confidence in themselves as a member of the group. It is a process that builds personal self-worth (Kurland, 1982). These have been used in the United States as well, sponsored by charitable groups such as the Kettering Foundation, to promote the discussion of topics related to public interest and concern (Oliver, 1990).

Service groups are an idea from the volunteering movement that is building momentum in the 21st century. This kind of group brings people together who might wish to combine their desire to do something for "those in need" with the interactive synergism of a group. A group might be organized around altruistic engagement or the opportunity for individuals within a group to combine their resources and engage the community in a context where helping others in need would be warranted. As noted in Chapter 7, there is systematic outcome data to support the effectiveness of altruistic intervention, and there is an emerging literature which suggests that altruism may be important in promoting positive aging.

COUNSELING OLDER ADULTS FROM SPECIAL POPULATIONS

Older adults are diverse with respect to gender, race, sexual orientation, and socioeconomic status; however, these characteristics have received little attention in counseling. The tendency to view the older client as predominantly white, male, heterosexual, and from the middle class is a subtle form of ageism that can create barriers to supportive services including mental health care (Braithwaite, 2002). A positive aging approach to counseling the elderly is sensitive to individual differences given that the everyday living concerns an older person might experience cannot always be addressed by a one-size-fits-all approach to counseling. But counseling can be tailored to address not only the chronological age of the person seeking help, but also gender, race, sexual orientation, or socioeconomic status. Examples of this complexity include, caregiving for an older gay man who is HIV positive (Altschuler, Katz, & Tynan, 2004), chronic depression in homeless women (Cohen, Ramirez, Teresi, Gallagher, & Sokolovsky, 1997), or whether an older Asian-American man will seek supportive counseling to deal with chronic pain following hip replacement surgery.

Gender

Over 60% of those over 65 years of age are women (U.S. Census, 2002). Although women are advantaged over men with respect to absolute longevity, women who live into very old age face a number of unique and difficult late-life issues. Foremost among these is the experience of widowhood. Demographic research suggests that women are nearly three times more likely to be widowed than similar-aged men (Murrell, Meeks, & Walker, 1991). Because widowhood can be an extremely stressful transition in old age, many women who lose a spouse to death report symptoms of chronic depression, poor health, and loneliness. In addition, older women who find themselves single in late life for a variety of reasons may suffer negative socioeconomic consequences, particularly if they have not pursued a career during the course of their life span. Those who have been employed outside the home may well have been paid less than men in the same job, and consequently retire with less money.

A positive aging approach to counseling is sensitive to whether the older female client feels disenfranchised from the mainstream of society, lonely, or powerless to change her situation. An example of a positive aging intervention is a group support therapy approach developed by Lorraine Gutierrez (1990) that brought together elderly African-American women who were experiencing a common issue; namely, caring for an impaired spouse or other loved one. In this instance, Gutierrez focused on African-American women because they are a group that does not typically seek professional counseling to help with their issues. The group therapy curriculum was based on three principles that Gutierrez described as central to the worldview of these women (2004). These principles were: (1) creating a shared group consciousness through storytelling; (2) teaching problem-solving skills specific to caregiving; and (3) helping group members develop personal advocacy skills to mobilize their coping resources. One of the goals of this group intervention was to help these women change their attributions that they were powerless to obtain resources from the larger community. Through a shared group format that focused on the collective power of the support group Gutierrez was able to create a sense of empowerment and hopefulness in these women that they could obtain support from the community to address many of their issues.

Race

Older adults are heterogeneous with respect to race. And, as the racial diversity of the United States increases, the characteristics of the typical elderly person who may need counseling is changing markedly. The 2000 U.S. Census reflected that of adults 65 years and older, 84% were white versus 16% who were an ethnic minority (defined as Black/African American, American Indian/Alaska Natives, Asian and Pacific Islander, and Hispanic). In 2030, this contrast is anticipated to change to 75% white versus 25% ethnic minority, and in 2050, 64% white versus 36% ethnic minority (Federal Interagency Forum on Aging Related Statistics [FIFARS], 2000; Brangman, et al., 2003; Panidya, 2005).

Research suggests that cultural values may produce barriers to accessing needed community services and that for the older ethnic minority adult who is seeking help, options for obtaining such assistance from outside their cultural group are limited (Sanchez-Ayendez, 1988). In this regard, the press to conform and to play a specific culturally defined role may be associated, for some, with conflict or animosity, particularly if there are services available in the community which they cannot access but that could otherwise address their concerns. It is easy to imagine the difficulties that are emergent in this kind of scenario. For example, for some older ethnic minority adults who are no longer able to drive and who must rely on public transportation, issues negotiating such travel in poor areas where crime rates are high, can put an older person at high risk for being victimized by crime. In addition, because many older, first generation ethnic minority adults often speak English poorly or are unable to speak or read English, such deficits may create barriers to goods and services, particularly if age-related disability restricts the older person's access to familiar areas for shopping, banking, and other community services.

A positive aging approach to older adults from ethnic minority groups should not only be sensitive to issues of access to services, professional assistance, and community support, but should also provide strategies to help a person deal with his or her concerns in ways that are culturally consistent. The extent to which traditional lifestyle behaviors influence coping should be understood. For example, an older bereaving Jamaican widow may benefit more in resolving her grief if a counselor helped her reconnect with her parish priest who could help her resolve her grief, versus an approach designed to alter maladaptive cognitions. An excellent example of positive aging in action for older ethnic minority adults is the El Portal Latino Alzheimer's Project, an interorganizational community-based collaborative project for dementia care services (Bailey & McNally, 1996). This approach to dementia care employs a collection of nonprofit groups sensitive to Spanish-speaking older adults who reside in California (Ranney, 2003). The Project provides, among other things, Spanish language adult daycare respite, in-home care, in-home food delivery services, as well as a range of advocacy and educational opportunities through in-person visits and telephone helplines. The El Portal Latino Alzheimer's Project attempts to create a "one-stop shopping" approach for services for Hispanic older adults. This is accomplished in a culturally relevant way from within the Hispanic community (Aranda, Villa, Trejo, Ramirez, & Ranney, 2003).

Sexual Orientation

Older gay, lesbian, and bisexual adults face special challenges in coping with life in contemporary society. Many of these older persons moved through adulthood with a same-sex sexual orientation and not surprisingly, a common theme for them is the social stigma and prejudice they may have experienced as a consequence of their same-sex orientation. Older gay and lesbian clients may have a number of age-related concerns including (1) caregivers desiring to gain access to their impaired loved one's medical records in order to make decisions about their partner's medical care; (2) gay and lesbian couples who have concerns about power of attorney, wills, and partner medical benefits; (3) older couples who have been estranged from one or both partners' families; and (4) relationship issues related to adult children.

In addition to the social issues noted above, awareness of the psychological concerns unique to gay, lesbian, and bisexual elderly adults have received attention only in recent years. In one national survey of a sample of nearly 2000 lesbian adults (Bradford, Caitlin, & Rothblum, 1994), 37% of those surveyed reported having been abused as an adult or child, 32% reported have been raped or attacked, and 19% had been involved in incestuous relationships earlier in life. A sizable number (30%) reported receiving mental health therapy in the past. Among the areas of concern for older lesbians, use of alcohol in old age was high and appeared to increase with age. Over one-third of lesbians 55 years and older reported that they were chronic cigarette smokers. Of the total group, older lesbians were the least likely to have openly declared their sexual orientation to family or friends. These statistics suggest that for older lesbians, issues related to their sexuality, their mood, and their relationships with others were of concern. However, of the total group, older lesbians were the least likely to seek counseling from professionals.

For older gay men, issues of stigma and prejudice are also prominent. It should be noted that for those persons 50 years and older, the mental health community treated their sexual orientation as a psychiatric disorder, and this stereotyping of their sexual orientation as a maladaptive life choice represented a substantial barrier for mental health treatment. An issue of particular concern for older gay men is sexually transmitted diseases including HIV/AIDS. It has been estimated that between 10 and 17% of U.S. AIDS cases occur in people over 50 years of age. Between 1990 and 2001 the number of AIDS cases in gay men 50 years and older exceeded 90,000 (U.S. Centers for Disease Control, 2002). There are several unique issues faced by older adults who are either at risk for AIDS/HIV or have been exposed to the disease. These include misdiagnosis, the stereotype that AIDS/HIV is a disease that only affects young people, poor medical management of the disease once it has been diagnosed, and a lack of education about ways to engage in safe sex practices to protect oneself from infection.

Therefore, an important area for positive aging counseling in older gay, lesbian, and bisexual persons is the development and dissemination of educational materials that are both accessible and meaningful to those who are over 50. An example of positive aging in relation to HIV/AIDS treatment and prevention in older adults is a model curriculum that several researchers developed for AIDS education specifically targeting older adults (Altschuler et al., 2004). In this study, a questionnaire was sent to several hundred older persons who self-reported that they were gay or lesbian. The information packet queried areas of interest and concern regarding AIDS education and prevention. From these participants three topics were identified and information was developed that addressed these areas. These are: (1) How is HIV/AIDS relevant to my life and situation? (2) How do I speak up about my concerns about AIDS/HIV to my health care provider? and (3) What are the ways that I can discuss my sexuality with people in my life including friends and family? These researchers then identified curricular materials that addressed these expressed concerns. In addition, they identified settings where AIDS education training would be most accessible to older persons including senior and community centers. They examined specific groups of older adults who would likely benefit from such education, and at the same time, who would be least likely to access educational programs.

This kind of approach to AIDS/HIV education and training—that considers the special needs facing older adults who are at risk for contracting AIDS/HIV—is an excellent example of positive aging in action, given that it is: (1) A proactive and systematic approach to finding a meaningful way to interact with older persons about the disease and the ways in which it can impact their lives. (2) It affirms the fact that older gay men adults are at risk for the disease and that their well-being is served when they learn how to protect themselves through safe sex practices. (3) It works to dispel harmful stereotypes that marginalize older gay men and proliferate misinformation about who is at risk and why.

For example, recent studies indicate that older heterosexual postmenopausal women are a subgroup of persons who are particularly vulnerable to sexually transmitted diseases (STDs). Gomez (2002) reported that this risk may be due, in part, to inadequate health education about STDs in these women for several reasons: (1) During the social era in which they lived their younger years, these women may have feared pregnancy more than STD risk. As they became post-menopausal, their risk of pregnancy was reduced freeing them to engage in unprotected heterosexual relationships. However, at the same time, as a group, they lacked awareness of the substantially increased prevalence of incurable STDs, including HIV/AIDS, that became apparent in the late 1980s. Because the risk for STDs is nearly four times higher for men than for women in this age group (Deneberg, 1997), unprotected sex puts this current cohort of post-menopausal women at even higher risk. Predictably, such women report poor access to and stereotypical fear of health services that can provide low cost or free STD testing. (2) Post-menopausal women may also view the symptoms of STDs (such as pelvic pain, heavy menstrual flow, and smelly vaginal discharge), as normative signs of old age. This kind of misperception is further evidence of the social stereotyping that has occurred in this age group leading to poor health awareness of normative reproductive changes versus disease processes in old age. Not understanding the nature of one's reproductive health may prevent older women who are sexually active from seeking regular diagnostic screening for STDs including HIV/AIDS, even if such screening is affordable. Gordon and Thompson (1995) estimated that older post-menopausal women are one-fifth as likely as their younger female counterparts to insist on condom use from a male sex partner. This underscores the need for proactive health-prevention strategies that target this vulnerable older female population.

Socioeconomic Issues

As a group, older adults have smaller incomes, are less able to move from their homes, have a higher incidence rate of chronic disease, and are more likely to need (but less able to afford) professional counseling services than younger persons. These and other issues may combine to make persons in late life vulnerable to socioeconomic hardships including poverty. In some cases this may be a new experience for an older person who has previously enjoyed the benefits of economic stability. However, the untimely death of a spouse, a major chronic illness, or a significant life change can create financial problems that are difficult if not impossible to recover from, particularly if a person is on a fixed-income or entirely dependent on social security. Older adults facing socioeconomic hardships for the first time in old age are at risk for mental health problems including depression and anxiety as well as social ostracism through homelessness.

The elderly make up a substantial percentage of those who are chronically homeless. It has been estimated that as high as 20% of homeless persons are 50 years of age and older (Kutza & Keigher, 1991). This group of poverty stricken chronically homeless persons is substantially different from older adults who have become impoverished for the first time due to negative circumstances in old age. Those who have been chronically homeless for their entire lives have a higher probability of having lifelong problems with mental illness and may also have long-standing patterns of drug addiction, criminal records, and a history of intermittent incarceration (Cohen, 1999). For these reasons, it is important to determine, through careful assessment, the circumstances under which an older person is in socioeconomic difficulty.

A positive aging approach to counseling an older person who is socioeconomically challenged and may also be struggling with mental health issues due to a lack of resources, is complex. For instance, the chronically homeless may need extended and ongoing assistance, including a coordinated system of specialized services that can meet their daily living needs, health and mental health-care needs, transportation assistance, and opportunities for developing skills for sustaining themselves in the community (Doolin, 1986). Counseling may be only a small part of this network of assistance. For those persons who have not had a lifelong experience with homelessness, but who find themselves economically challenged in old age, there may be a number of informal resources that can be harnessed, including extended family, neighbors, and friends (Crane, 1999). The older person who has previously lived in a middle-class context will often have access to social and community resources including church, senior center, community service organization, and social groups.

CONCLUDING COMMENTS

Mental health issues are a reality in old age just as they are across earlier periods of the life span. In this chapter two common psychiatric disorders were highlighted; depression and anxiety. Although only a small percentage of older adults would qualify for such diagnoses, the symptoms of these disorders are likely to be encountered by most people at some time during late life. Older adults are vulnerable to specific events that could bring on these symptoms including age-related cognitive decline, loss of social support, role changes, and a decline in available resources. Several approaches to counseling were described in this chapter that are supported by empirical data that indicate they are effective in addressing older adult concerns and can promote positive aging: psychodynamic therapy, cognitive behavioral therapy, family systems therapy, and existential therapy (including life review). In addition to how these therapy approaches work, this chapter described different ways that therapy can be delivered including individual and group formats. Finally, the role of sociocultural differences, including gender, ethnicity, and sexual orientation were presented as examples of factors that are important to consider if the goal is to make therapy meaningful and of value to the broader cross section of older persons who represent individual and cultural diversity.

Chapter 7

POSITIVE SPIRITUALITY AND MEANING-BASED COUNSELING

How can personal meaning be useful in counseling the aged? This is a challenging question because it underscores the fact that many of the traditional approaches to therapy were not conceived with the older adult in mind (Hepple, 2004). For this reason, there could be aspects of these approaches that may not be perceived as meaningful (or even relevant) to the older adult. This issue was echoed by Antonucci (2000) in her presidential address to the Gerontological Society of America: "As we find ways to improve the lives of older people and ameliorate the diseases which afflict them, we are also confronted by the reality that we are often unable to successfully utilize these discoveries" (p. 5).

The meaning-based life-span concepts that are discussed in this chapter take into account belief systems or ideologies that generate an inherently positive bias in how one views the world. Take for instance the notion of religious beliefs and how these influence a person's perceptions of the world as well as the meaning ascribed to circumstances that shape the outcome of living. Although not everyone endorses a religious ideology or a personal religious belief, the concept of religion is a pervasive theme in the American culture (Gallup & Lindsay, 1999). A Gallup poll estimated that over 65% of Americans considered themselves religious (Gallup, 1985) and over 82% acknowledged a personal need for spiritual growth (Gallup &

Jones, 2000). Religion, then, might be an area to begin the search for meaning-based concepts that would have relevance to counseling older adults who are striving to be positive agers.

There is a growing body of evidence which suggests that concepts embedded in religious beliefs or spirituality are positively associated with health (Miller & Thoresen, 2003), although how religious beliefs enhance health is poorly understood. In their review of the health benefits of a religious or a spiritual orientation, Powell and her colleagues reported that one's personal belief system can be construed as a general protective factor that prevents the development of disease in people who are otherwise healthy (Powell, Shahabi, & Thoresen, 2003). What appears to be the case for disease prevention, however, is that one's belief system as it manifests itself in observable behavior tends to enhance one's sense of well-being. For example, when a person's religious beliefs motivate them to attend church and socialize with others or engage in religious activities such as helping those in need, the consequences of such behavior have the potential to reduce the risk of disease and enhance longevity (Thoresen, 2003).

Older adults are the most likely group to consider their religious beliefs an important resource in coping with the challenges and difficulties of living. And the concept of religious belief has recently been described in the scientific literature as one source of positive aging (Crowther et al., 2002). Crowther and her colleagues have suggested that the term *positive spirituality* could be put forward as a concept to clarify this domain of meaning with respect to better understanding the dimensionality of positive aging. They note that *positive spirituality* is "a developing and internalized personal relation with the sacred or transcendent [that] promotes the wellness and the welfare of self and others. . . . Positive [spirituality] provide[s] a cognitive framework that reduces stress and increases purpose and meaning" (p. 614).

Their conception of positive spirituality is distinct from terms like *religion* or *spirituality*. Specifically, *positive spirituality* is not bound by an organized system of beliefs, practices, or doctrines that would be descriptive of religion; nor is it restricted to the personal quest for ultimate understanding that would be characteristic of spirituality. Instead, it focuses on the individual's inherent motivation toward self-improvement (or enhancing the welfare of others) as a way to broaden one's own value in the present and in the future in personal and social processes for the promotion of "good" in the world.

Positive spirituality, then, is a term that allows for further exploration of meaning-based concepts that could be embedded in religious ideologies or spiritual quests that are also part of psychological and developmental theories of aging. Meaning-based life-span strategies consistent with positive spirituality can be found in the developmental theories described earlier; namely, Erikson's life stages theory, continuity theory, and SOC. The power of strategies that use personal meaning as the active ingredient of intervention, such as altruism, have been described from a religious perspective and in the psychological theories noted above. These concepts are also embedded in contemporary definitions of growing old including positive aging.

From the MacArthur Foundation Research Network on Aging (Albert et al., 1995; Berkman et al., 1993; Seeman et al., 1994) Rowe and Kahn (1998) drew several important conclusions about the defining characteristics of aging that could be used in developing meaning-based counseling interventions: "If successful aging is to be more than the imitation of youth, however, we must also ask whether there are valued human attributes that increase with age, or that might do so under appropriate conditions of opportunity and encouragement" (p. 139). This quotation emphasizes that although positive spirituality, like other developmental life-span characteristics (such as wisdom), are not necessarily guaranteed if one simply manages to live into old age, the unique conditions and processes of adult aging are essential prerequisites to acquiring such skills or attributes in later life. There are personalized aspects of the fully developed older adult that must be understood and acted upon with respect to positive aging. Every older person is a complex human being with a history of strategies for dealing with the issues of living and if these aspects of the person are not acknowledged or ignored by the counselor, well-intentioned interventions will not be perceived as useful or meaningful to the older client.

There is a growing scientific literature that suggests there are certain thematic life-span characteristics which, if developed, can powerfully facilitate positive aging (Antonucci, 2000; Dulin et al. 2001; McCullough, Emmons, & Tsang, 2000). With respect to labeling these concepts, the term *meaning-based* should be emphasized. Several of these meaning-based concepts have been found in the empirical literature to promote health and well-being including forgiveness, altruism, and gratitude. Each of these concepts is tied to a specific source of meaning acquired during the course of living. Forgiveness facilitates relationships; altruism establishes purpose; and gratitude is a source of positive emotion. These meaning-based life span strategies, then, have utility for addressing a range of issues in late life including age-related decline, loss of a loved one to death, caregiving, life transitions such as retirement, and end-of-life concerns.

It is important to note that these meaning-based life-span strategies may seem as though they are very personal in nature, and the reader might link them to organized religion. They are, however, more generally associated with the acquired ability to integrate experiences across life in the pursuit of understanding how to best get along in the world and how to help others in the process. These meaning-based concepts will be defined with respect to their epistemological roots and how they fit within the previously described theories of aging, including SOC, continuity theory, and Erikson's life stages, as well as their connection to positive aging.

FORGIVENESS: A WORKING DEFINITION

From a religious perspective, forgiveness has been defined in various ways. From a philosophical–religious perspective forgiveness involves absolving oneself of negative feelings toward someone who has offended, and replacing them with a compassionate response (Witvliet, 2001). North (1987) has suggested that compassion requires that the forgiver "view the wrongdoer with mercy, benevolence, and love while recognizing that he has willfully abandoned his right to them" (p. 502). From a sociopsychological perspective forgiveness has been operationalized as the propensity of a person to let go of resentment and negative judgments toward an offender. In this sense, forgiveness is the skill or capability to reframe negative feelings that are directed toward an offender with emotions that evoke compassion and generosity (Enright, 1991, Enright & Coyle, 1994).

Forgiveness is often associated with spiritual and emotional healing. In fact, across all of the major world religions forgiveness, as a religious tenet, has been deemed not only essential to a healthy spiritual life, but prerequisite to salvation (Rye et al., 2000). In contemporary psychological literature, forgiveness has also been linked to physical healing and well-being (Krause & Ellison, 2003).

In the field of pastoral counseling, forgiveness plays an important role in healing emotional wounds (Brandsma, 1982). A number of strategies have emerged from pastoral counseling where forgiveness has been a central part of therapeutic strategy. In the contemporary psychological literature, the concept of forgiveness (sometimes termed *letting go*) has been utilized to address a wide variety of psychological maladies including loneliness, social phobia, anger, and bereavement. Forgiveness is prominent in a number of behavior change programs including the Alcoholics Anonymous (AA) 12-step program (detailed below) that embodies a spiritual process of forgiveness as part of the recovery from alcoholism (Mackenzie & Allen, 2003):

Step 1: The admission that one is powerless over alcohol
Step 2: Belief that a power greater than ourselves can restore us
Step 3: Decision to turn our will and our lives over to God
Step 4: A moral inventory of ourselves
Step 5: Admit to God, to ourselves, and to others our wrongs
Step 6: Be ready to have God remove all these defects
Step 7: Ask God to remove our shortcomings
Step 8: Emotionally make amends to all those we have harmed
Step 9: Act to correct all the wrongs we have done
Step 10: When we are wrong, admit it
Step 11: Pray and meditate to improve our contact with God
Step 12: Experience a spiritual awakening from following these steps

The 12-step AA program utilizes among other change strategies, values clarification on the part of the recovering alcoholic with the goal of developing a spiritual approach to living that is incompatible with alcohol abuse. An important attitudinal and behavioral component of the AA model is the seeking of (and finding) forgiveness as described in steps 8 (make amends to all those we have harmed), 9 (act to correct all the wrongs we have done), and 10 (when we are wrong admit it). AA is a concrete example of how principles of forgiveness can be a component of a general approach to life change that is designed to correct maladaptive behavior (Poage, Ketzenberger, & Olson, 2004); however, there is growing scientific interest in the utilization of forgiveness concepts in psychological interventions to promote well-being across the life span and in old age (Enright & Fitzgibbons, 2000; Hebl & Enright, 1993).

Given the possibility that forgiveness may be a meaning-based life span skill that can promote positive aging in later life irregardless of a person's circumstances or belief system, the first step in utilizing forgiveness as a treatment strategy is to operationalize it as a life skill coping strategy.

An important aspect of forgiveness requires understanding how the propensity to forgive emerges and matures across the life span. For many people, forgiveness is learned very early in life, within the context of organized religion or taught within the nuclear family as a way to promote familial harmony. From this early introduction, forgiveness is reinforced as a part of everyday living skills. Children can learn at a very early age the powerful reparative properties of acknowledging to another person their sorrow at having engaged in an offensive behavior, or the experience of accepting an apology from someone who has wronged them.

Even in the secular educational system, how well one gets along with others at school often depends on how well the concept of forgiveness is understood. It is safe to assume that, if queried about forgiveness, no member of contemporary society would be unaware of the concept or what it means, although there would be great variations with respect to how strongly people believe in the efficacy of forgiveness, as well as how many practice this life skill in their daily lives.

Although a relatively easy concept to grasp intellectually, forgiveness can be difficult to master. The ability to forgive a wrongdoer, to forgive oneself, or to forgive God or nature requires one to subjugate self-needs and personal defensiveness. So, it is not surprising that people range widely in their capacity to forgive. Researchers have even developed treatment manuals to train people how to improve their forgiveness skills. In one study, forgiveness was conceptualized as a skill set that could be taught through a 17-unit curriculum consisting of one-hour classes (Freedman & Enright, 1996). The goal of forgiveness training in this instance was to help incest survivors learn to forgive their perpetrators and through this process experience better psychological well-being as a consequence. The topics for this forgiveness course included: learning to examine one's own defense mechanisms in the process of adapting to being wronged; the management of and appropriate expression of one's anger associated with the wrongful act; understanding shame and guilt that occurs when one is wronged; learning how to express emotion about a wrongdoing; the role of forgiveness in helping to reframe one's feelings toward a wrongful act and the wrongdoer; committing oneself to forgive even when it is not possible to physically right a wrongful act or receive an apology from the wrongdoer; understanding the underlying processes of forgiving including empathy; learning to view the world as an imperfect place, and recognizing (as well as accepting) positive emotions when these return as a consequence of forgiving. As part of this study, a manualized version of this curriculum was utilized (Enright, 1991).

With respect to the person who has been wronged, forgiveness can bring a sense of peace and well-being, even if the wrongdoer never seeks such forgiveness from the offended person. It is generally believed by most people that the capacity to forgive is within every individual who has been wronged (Gartner, 1988), and that one often learns how to forgive by forgiving another for a wrong deed, even though the offender never acknowledges that a wrong has been done. So, as a life skill, the ability to forgive combines a sense that it is important to live and act in such a way as to not harm other people, but also without remorse, to let go of situations and others who have offended.

The Function of Forgiveness in Counseling

In applying forgiveness as a counseling strategy with older adults, four criteria should be utilized: (1) describing and depersonalizing the wrong deed; (2) putting the wrong deed in a life-span perspective; (3) finding peace of mind through a focus on the present and future; (4) reframing the event as a learning/growth experience—a source of positive aging.

Forgiveness is effective for relationship or intrapersonal issues where the individual is unable to let go of a poor decision or a personal life error or is living a lifestyle that is inconsistent with his or her core value system. Thus, forgiveness may only require a change of heart or a new way of looking at an old problem for healing to occur. This is highlighted in the vignette that follows:

> Sarah was a 77-year-old widow who lived alone, although she did have one adult daughter who lived in another state. Sarah was haunted by the memory that the day before her husband unexpectedly died of a stroke they had engaged in a somewhat bitter argument. The context of the argument was: Sarah wanted to drive out to see her daughter the next week for her daughter's birthday. Sarah's husband, Bill, on the other hand, preferred to fly their daughter to their home and celebrate their daughter's birthday in their home. Although Sarah's daughter was willing to celebrate her birthday at either location, Sarah and Bill were both determined "to have their way." Unfortunately, their argument went on into the evening and they went to bed upset at one another. During the night, Sarah heard her husband groaning. When she tried to wake him up, he was delirious and spoke incoherently. She immediately called an ambulance. When the paramedics arrived, they indicated to Sarah that her husband had experienced a severe stroke that had taken his life. She was devastated by this event and blamed their argument for precipitating her husband's stroke, and because of it she felt unable to stop her grieving process.

Sarah's experience represents one of those chance events that can leave a permanent scar on an otherwise positive set of memories. In this instance, Sarah's marriage to her husband, Bill, could be characterized as having been stable and positive. There was every indication that it was a source of strength and well-being for both individuals. Certainly, it was not a marriage without some difficulties and arguments. But, it is unlikely that Bill's stroke was directly connected to their situational argument. However, Sarah was left with a lingering sense of guilt around the circumstances leading up to Bill's death. Psychological relief could possibly be found in reinterpreting the event from a more forgiving perspective. While attending a widow support group that was sponsored by the local funeral home, Sarah made an appointment with a grief counselor to work on her unresolved issue.

A forgiveness intervention might proceed in the following way: Help Sarah to reframe the event. It might be useful to encourage her to consider their argument as a sign that they had a healthy disagreement and that their marriage was such that they both felt free to discuss their different points of view with each other. Encourage Sarah to recount other arguments that she had with Bill across their life. Arguments were not uncommon, and it may be, from a life-span perspective that there would have been even more had Bill continued to live. It was unfortunate about the timing of this argument, and had it been a week (or a month) before his stroke, Sarah would likely have made no direct connection between the two.

A forgiveness approach to counseling would help Sarah search for peace of mind. She might do this by imagining how Bill would view her reaction to their fight, should he still be alive. In this instance, the goal would be to help Sarah identify how to forgive herself through manipulating the memory of her husband. Since it is not possible to go back into the past and relive the experience, only in the present can she rework the event. If she is religious she might put the matter in God's hands. If she is not religious, it might be in the context of a life-learning experience; that is, how can this loss help you to become a more adaptive person in the future. What can Sarah learn about herself and her needs as a result of reflecting on this event?

This example of a forgiveness intervention focuses on self-forgiveness. This is often one of the more prevalent concerns that adults experience in later life, particularly as they reflect back on past relationships. It is a human propensity for some to focus on the negative at the expense of the positive in intimate relationships. The power of forgiveness is to give people permission to let go of negative memories and through this process find peace of mind. It should be noted that processes underlying a forgiveness intervention are applicable with respect to the other two relational domains as well; namely, forgiveness of others and forgiveness from nature (or God).

Psychotherapy research with older clients has also produced positive outcomes when forgiveness has been employed as part of the therapeutic treatment. In one study, a forgiveness intervention was employed with a group of 24 elderly women who had reported that they were victims of wrongdoing for a variety of reasons (Hebl & Enright, 1993). In this study an eight-week course in forgiveness yielded improvement in well-being in this group of elderly women over a control group. Specifically, those who received forgiveness training felt less hatred and anger toward their identified wrongdoers and a greater willingness to help others as a consequence. This study and others like it (Enright & Fitzgibbons, 2000) suggest that forgiveness training can be a useful meaning-based strategy for promoting psychological health in old age and may be as effective for promoting positive aging in later life in persons suffering from depression and anxiety (associated with feeling victimized by others) as more traditional psychotherapeutic approaches.

ALTRUISM: A WORKING DEFINITION

Altruism embodies unselfish acts for the benefit of others (Post, Underwood, Schloss, & Hurlbut 2002). Like forgiveness, altruism is often articulated as a component of a religious belief system espoused as a way to promote well-being in others and in oneself.

From a psychological perspective, psychoanalytic theorists such as Alfred Adler characterized altruism as involving a process associated with feelings of self-worth and personal meaning through a focus away from the self and toward others (Adler, 1937). The Adlerian notion of altruism is associated with positive life adjustment and a greater sense of purpose in life. Dulin and colleagues (Dulin, Hill, Anderson, & Rasenussen, 2001) examined life satisfaction in over 100 low-income older adult volunteers who were identified as participants in the Foster Grandparent/Senior Companion program in Salt Lake City, Utah. The Senior Companion Program is a federally-funded program employing older adult volunteers who serve the frail elderly in a variety of contexts such as assisting with household chores and financial management. Foster Grandparents provided services to children and adolescents who were in poor economic and social circumstances. To be eligible to participate in these programs, these older volunteers must be, by definition, below the poverty line in income. The time spent volunteering was a minimum of 10 hours per week. On several measures of life satisfaction, including the Life Satisfaction in the Elderly Scale (LSES; Salamon & Conte, 1984), that assesses life satisfaction across six domains, including meaning, social contacts, mood, self-concept, health, and finances, their scores on this instrument were impressive as compared to a national normative sample (see Figure 7.1), Although these volunteers acknowledged that they were poor with respect to finances and less healthy than the typical American citizen over 60 years of age, they scored high on this instrument. In fact, their LSES scores on meaning, social contacts, mood, and self-concept were better than a normative sample of middle-income older adults who were not engaged in volunteer activities.

Because altruism can take many forms, the focus here is limited to its behavioral manifestation; that is, acts of helping (or service) to others without the expectation of personal gain. In this regard, philanthropy, volunteerism, and caregiving would all embody altruistically motivated help-giving. In older adults, studies in the scientific literature have produced consistent evidence in support of the beneficial properties of altruistic help giving (Morrow-Howell,

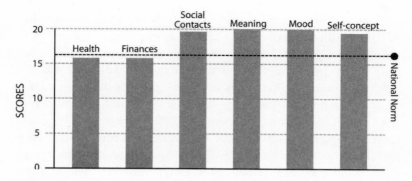

FIGURE 7.1. LIFE SATISFACTION ACROSS SIX DOMAINS (LSES). (SALOMON & CONTE, 1986; ADAPTED FROM DULIN ET AL., 2001).

et al., 2003; Van Willigen, 2000). A group of older adults who were volunteers in a community context assisting low-income families were studied (Kuehne & Sears, 1993). The nature of their volunteer work consisted of providing direct assistance to families who were raising children with a chronic illness. The researchers found that, in this group of older volunteers, the act of helping was strongly associated with enhanced life satisfaction in these older volunteers.

One explanation for the beneficial effects of volunteering may be that it represents a way to replace lost sources of meaning that have previously been attached to established roles earlier in adulthood (such as one's occupation). In one study that involved nearly 400 persons from the National Survey of Midlife Development in the United States (MIDUS; Greenfield & Marks, 2004), researchers found that those older persons who indicated that they were volunteers reported better well-being than those who were not volunteering. In examining the mechanism underlying this finding, it was discovered that the extent to which a person was able to replace previous formal life roles with volunteerism, greater well-being ensued. Other studies have found that volunteering engenders positive emotions (Bond, 1982) and that those who consistently volunteer have a greater likelihood of living longer than nonvolunteers (Musick et al., 1999; Oman, Thoresen, & McMahon, 1999).

Such research suggests that altruistically motivated helping may serve to buffer an older adult against many of the common vicissitudes of aging. From the point of view of a counseling strategy, altruistic helping may have properties that can actualize psychological resources and promote positive aging.

Altruism in Counseling

Of the meaning-based life-span strategies described previously, altruism is, perhaps, the most concrete. To engage in an altruistic intervention requires only that the person identify a worthwhile volunteer task to undertake. Once this has been done, the client can begin the process of volunteering, which should then produce some positive consequences with respect to emotional health. However, if a person does not have a life history of serving others it may be important to encourage the client to develop a help-giving mindset. The idea that one might be able to get psychological relief by helping others might seem counterintuitive, but below are several ideas that might be used to catalyze an attitude conducive to altruistic behavioral lifestyle routines.

- Encourage the client to think of him- or herself as someone who has worth or value. As this occurs, identify those instances in the past when the client's value was manifest in the act of helping.
- Have the client recollect when he or she has helped other people in need and how this made the client feel.
- Explore with the client contexts or situations where the client perceives that help-giving behaviors might make a difference.
- Encourage the client to begin a help-giving routine to reap the benefits of these helping behaviors with respect to the recipient, as well as the client.

Altruism requires action as is highlighted in the vignette that follows:

Maria was a 69-year-old widow who lived alone and was becoming frail with the passage of time. She was a wealthy woman who had devoted her whole life to a career in finance, and she had hoped to retire, travel, and benefit from all of her hard-earned dollars. She was a driven professional and worked into her mid-60s. At the point of retirement from her firm, Maria, at her annual physical exam, was diagnosed with a form of macular degeneration, a degenerative eye disease that she was told would produce blindness over the course of a few years. Maria was devastated; she could no longer follow her life plan. In fact, the progressive nature of her eye disease left her mostly homebound within two years. She began to obsessively worry about her health and her money. When she was younger she had benefited from psychotherapy that focused on a relationship issue, so she thought it would be useful to seek out counseling at this time to assist her in coping with her lifestyle restrictions and the burden associated with these. In her first session with a licensed professional counselor, he raised the possibility that the source of her current emotional pain was less related to her eye disease and more to her intense self-focus and worry. Together, they discussed ways that Maria could change her self-focus. One that came to mind and that appealed to Maria was volunteering as a phone counselor for older adults with macular degeneration who, like her, needed contact, but were homebound. The counselor put Maria in touch with this service organization. She received the necessary training and began spending about five hours per week contacting patients. It was not long before Maria's resilience returned. She became very enthusiastic about her volunteer experience, and made several new friends in the process. Although she continued to worry about her health and her finances, the obsessive nature of these worries diminished over time.

This vignette emphasizes how easily an altruistic counseling intervention can be engaged. Although the concept of utilizing volunteerism as an intervention to enhance well-being has been recommended by self-help authors for decades and theological scholars for centuries, a specific counseling strategy that engages help-giving as an intervention for promoting positive aging of the helper has not been articulated in the treatment literature. The impact of altruistically motivated help-giving, as a way of developing peace of mind, can be foundational in moving the focus of psychological resources from self-concerns to a more outward concern for the welfare of others.

GRATITUDE: A WORKING DEFINITION

Gratitude is a positive emotion that is connected to appreciation for the "good things" in life, while at the same time recognizing that life can sometimes be difficult and challenging. For many, the ups and downs of living can only be appreciated if one is able to cultivate gratitude for the privilege of living with both the pleasures and challenges of life. Thus, in a sense, gratitude is the belief that although the world is not perfect, an attitude of "thankfulness" can be a source of well-being and peace of mind. It has been suggested that it is impossible to be both grateful and miserable simultaneously. This is likely because gratitude requires the explicit acknowledgment that life is worthwhile regardless of the difficulty of a person's circumstances.

However, to interpret gratitude as only a mood state, less accessible to conscious awareness, highlights the notion that gratitude is a consequence rather than a determinant of adaptation. Like forgiveness, and altruism, a grateful disposition can also be construed as a life skill that a person learns in order to more optimally adapt to the challenges of living. Thus, gratitude could be operationalized for therapy purposes as a goal-directed emotion that can effect attentional processes to focus on ways to maximize quality of living irregardless of external context or circumstances. Grateful people learn how to experience positive aging even when facing difficult challenges or problems.

This definition of gratitude suggests that it is primarily a cognitive (or attitudinal) skill. To feel grateful for something or someone requires simply thinking about that person (or thing) in a positive way. In fact, as is portrayed in the vignette below, one can construct grateful feelings in circumstances that might not usually engender it.

Deborah was an energetic middle-aged woman who ran a small laundry business in a large Eastern city. She enjoyed being in business for herself; however, recently, she had been required to sell her property to the City Planning Commission so that a new freeway could be built through the area. Although relocating her business seemed like an impossible task, she did sell her property, and moved to another part of the city. In the first year of her relocated business, she lost a considerable amount of money and had to take out a second mortgage on her home; eventually, she lost the business. Although this was a hardship, Deborah always kept an upbeat disposition with the following thought, "I am grateful that I had the chance to start my own business and, although it eventually failed, I was able to stay in business longer than I had ever imagined that I could." She had great pride around three awards that she had received from the Chamber of Commerce acknowledging her early success in starting a business.

Deborah had every reason to feel bitter and resentful. She was clearly a victim of difficult circumstances; however, her expression of gratitude acknowledged that she was aware that life does deal out challenges to everyone from time to time. The easy thing to do is to express negativity, worry, and resentment. In fact, most observers would feel that Deborah would be justified in being angry, bitter, and resentful, particularly since it may be that she had been wronged by the planning commission. Gratitude does not mean that a person does not advocate or assert him- or herself. However, if the goal is optimal adaptation to an inevitable loss and the emotional consequences of such a loss, a possible approach to coping would be to cultivate gratitude for the "silver linings" in any otherwise negative event. Gratitude, in this sense, can be engaged as a source for positive aging and, can be applied to maintain a positive mindset, even when conditions or situations take a turn for the worse.

Gratitude in Counseling

Emmons and McCollough (2003), conducted a gratitude intervention that consisted of the following instructions provided to their participants for beginning a journaling process: "There are many things in our lives, both large and small, that we might be grateful about. Think back over the past week and write down on the lines below up to five things in your life that you are grateful or thankful for" (p. 388).

In their study, the participants who engaged in gratitude journaling showed heightened well-being across standardized measures of self-esteem and life satisfaction. Emmons and McCollough concluded that the primary effect of inducing feelings of gratitude through journaling was to generate positive emotional and interpersonal feelings. This study suggested that a counseling intervention that infuses "gratitude training" into its scheme will result in positive affect.

Below are several ideas for helping an older client generate a sense of gratitude.

1. Encourage the client to develop a gratitude journal. This involves recording thoughts during the day that are evidence of gratitude (reflecting on things that make a client smile, bring happiness or joy, or bring about feelings of peace).

Set a minimum number of entries per day (e.g., no less than five) and then encourage the client to systematically increase the number of entries. Review the gratitude journal during the course of each counseling session. Help the client learn to express, verbally, feelings of gratitude.

2. Help the client recollect when he or she felt grateful in the past. Explore how those feelings of gratitude influenced the quality of everyday living.

3. Help the client understand that the world is not perfect. Gratitude can be cultivated whether one is sick or healthy. Gratitude can be found in difficult situations. It may not solve a problem, but it can help a person find positives even when they may not be apparent.

The death of a loved one is a profoundly sorrowful event and the loss of such a relationship is not reversible. However, statements like, "I'm grateful for the time we had together," or "She lived a long and healthy life," can mediate negative emotions such as anger, sorrow, blame, guilt, and shame that might be associated with such a loss.

Gratitude can be a very accessible intervention adjunct because it primarily involves shifting one's state of mind. However, it does require practice and repetition in order for it to become a natural reaction to a negative life challenge. Further, gratitude is not an excuse for avoiding a problem or difficulty. In fact, the essence of gratitude is to generate emotional reserves that can then be used to tackle the problem with a new perspective or viewpoint that might make it more solvable.

A gratitude journal can encourage a client to practice thinking grateful thoughts even when a situation is such that the person has very little capability of changing. The end of life can be powerfully affected by the cultivation of gratitude on the part of the dying person, as well as those who are grieving the death of a loved one. Gratitude can also be applied in helping a person deal with more minor life transitions, such as the one described in the vignette that follows:

> Richard was a 66-year-old retiree who returned to college to get a second bachelor's degree in English. It was not long before he found himself struggling in several of his classes. In one class in particular, his professor made a number of negative comments on a paper he had written and the professor indicated that Richard needed to do some remedial work on his writing skills. The professor even went so far as to suggest that

Richard consider going to the campus counseling center to seek some guidance regarding his poor attitude toward the class. Richard, a professional person who worked for years as a technical writer was dumbfounded by this suggestion. He did, however, make an appointment with a counselor to discuss what he described as his problem with how to deal with an unreasonable and narrow-minded professor. For two sessions, Richard complained about this unreasonable professor and his frustrations with him, both in the class and when he got feedback about his papers. One of the interventions the counselor recommended that Richard engage in was a *gratitude journal*. The counselor suggested that Richard begin to think about reasons he was grateful to be attending this particular English class. Richard followed the counselor's advice and soon began to report that, although the class was difficult and he didn't agree with the professor, there was still much to be learned in this class. He was particularly grateful for his fellow students who were always supportive when Richard presented his work orally. Richard also reported that he was grateful to be learning to write differently from the way he had while working in industry, and he was impressed with how different the writing was in an academic context. Soon, Richard reported enjoying the class and even challenging the professor once or twice. He noted, "If I ever challenged my boss with new ideas, he would have fired me; however, even if the professor disagrees with my point of view it always ends up becoming an interesting classroom discussion."

This vignette highlights the power of cultivating a grateful attitude. The steps that Richard took to deal with this situation were: He let go of his sense of entitlement about writing. He placed positive value on his learning experience. He reframed his animosity toward the professor by changing his assumptions about the professor's motivations. He found a way to have fun with the experience. He diminished its seriousness. He found ways to build his self-confidence ("I can come up with new ideas").

Cultivating strong skills in developing a grateful disposition can protect a person against the numerous instances in life where injustice might occur. McCullough et al. (2002) suggested that people vary in gratitude across several dimensions including *intensity*—the strength of feeling grateful; *frequency*—how often a person can feel grateful; *density*—how many people one can be grateful to in a single event.

When asked, "Tom to whom are you grateful for getting a good education?" a rating high on "gratitude intensity" would be Tom's deep expressed appreciation (with emotion) for those who helped him versus a low gratitude intensity response that would simply recognize those who helped him. A rating high on "gratitude frequency" would be Tom's desire to share his gratitude with others whenever or wherever he could, versus a low gratitude frequency response where Tom would express gratitude only to a single person at one point in time. A rating high on "gratitude density" would be for Tom to identify many people including parents, friends, teachers, and informal mentors who helped him versus a low "gratitude density" response that might be reflected in Tom having difficulty thinking of people beyond his teachers for whom he was grateful for his education.

These gratitude dimensions may be useful in developing a counseling intervention that involves gratitude. The psychological literature suggests that gratitude is skill-based; that is, people can learn to be grateful through experience and practice. By providing a context in which a client can cultivate gratitude, a counselor can help a person build an important skill for preserving positive aging even when the inevitable challenges of living arise.

CONCLUDING COMMENTS

Well-intentioned counseling interventions frequently fail because they are not consistent with the kinds of coping strategies that an older adult may have developed across a full life span. This chapter has presented some novel approaches to change and adaptation that could be useful as counseling and psychotherapy adjuncts with respect to models of positive aging. Life-span skills such as forgiveness, altruism, and gratitude consider the whole person as actively shaping his or her world. This chapter has provided both a conceptual and empirical argument that these meaning-based life-span strategies are useful tools for dealing with some of the more difficult issues facing older adults. With respect to theory, SOC highlights each of these meaning-based concepts with the idea that they develop across the life span. Although a person may be exposed to these concepts at a very early age, the mature manifestation of forgiveness, altruism, and gratitude in repairing a relationship or reconciling personal loss can enhance quality of life as well as the well-being of those with whom the person is involved. Erikson's ideas underscore the notion that at each life stage the individual must resolve tensions between the self and society. These life-span skills can help in the resolution of such crises as well as foster increased maturity in the process. Meaning-based life-span skills can help to optimize the inevitable declines experienced in old age, promoting, as an outcome, positive aging.

Chapter 8

POSITIVE AGING IN PHYSICAL DISABILITY AND CAREGIVING

THE EMERGENCE OF CHRONIC disability and its consequences in old and very old age can represent discontinuities that have broad consequences, including the loss of independent living skills, and in its more advanced stages, the loss of the ability to handle self-care. Not only is disability problematic from a functional point of view, but it also can have serious psychological consequences including depression, anxiety, and a general sense of hopelessness about the future. For those older persons living with partners, the effect of a loved-one's physical and or cognitive disability can have a profound impact on quality of life due to the caregiving issues that emerge from such a situation. And although it is a normative part of very old age, anticipating that one will experience chronic disease significant enough to impair functioning can be anxiety provoking. The fact that those 85 years and older suffer from at least one disabling medical condition (Manton et al., 1997) suggests that developing coping strategies to address long-term disability are essential to the maintenance of well-being and life satisfaction. Given these issues, a psychological construct such as positive aging can be useful in helping older people cope with significant disability-related impairment.

What may be the case, however, is that positive aging will manifest itself in somewhat different ways than when a person's faculties or interpersonal relationships are intact. A person with a chronic disability may live in a residential care facility where choice is more restricted, access to the outside world is limited, and care is delivered by professionals as opposed to family and loved ones. In this respect, positive aging may be more focused on sustaining the person's selective independence within the dimensions of such a living context.

AGING AND DISABILITY

As people grow older, chronic health conditions tend to increase along with the physical and psychological symptoms associated with such conditions. Fries and Crapo (1981) have argued that although chronic disease is present in human physiology from birth, for all persons, the signs of disease are not discernible until the symptoms cross a "clinical" threshold. This is because the youthful body is able to compensate for disease and other deteriorative processes by accessing reserve capacity (see Chapter 2). Because very little reserve capacity remains in old age, compensation for the wear and tear of living is diminished, and for this reason even small accidents, such as a fall, can precipitate a chronic disabling condition. Even in the absence of accident or trauma, decline in organ strength, such as the heart and lungs, as well as general physiological function, such as the elasticity of the skin and strength of the bones, make an older person vulnerable to disability. Further, given that the underlying cause of disability is disease, chronic disability produces a number of serious life consequences that become worse as one gets older: reduced mobility, increased risk for accidents at home and lapses in self-care, all leading to the risk of loss of quality of life.

With respect to a working definition of age-related disability, Verbrugge and Jette (1994) suggest that it has two distinct features (pp. 4–5): (1) It emerges from chronic health conditions and can affect any activity from instrumental activities of daily living (i.e., household chores) to basic self-care activities (i.e., dressing and bathing). (2) The essential feature of disability involves difficulty in performing these kinds of activities in an everyday context and without help from another person (e.g., not being able to get out of bed without assistance).

With respect to age-related factors, two additional features should be added to this definition: (1) Disability, as it emerges in old age, is subject to age-related decline. Most disability in old age will get worse as the person grows older. (2) In very old age, people may have more than one disability that must be managed simultaneously, increasing the difficulty of coping with any single disability (Ostir et al., 1999).

Disability comes in many forms and there are a number of risk factors for chronic disability that can interact with chronological age and disease to accelerate deterioration. Such factors include physiological decline in cognitive and sensory function, lifestyle behaviors such as diet, smoking, and alcohol use, as well as social features such as lack of adequate social support and poor access to health care. If a person is obese, for example, this condition can speed the progression of chronic disability in old age. If an older person is economically poor and has minimal access to the health-care system, this can increase the extent to which disability will impair everyday functioning. The vignette below illustrates how chronic disability might impact everyday functioning.

Manuel, a 72-year-old Mexican American male had lived in South Los Angeles for all of his adult life. Manuel was an immigrant from Mexico and worked as a field hand in the California orange groves for many years. He had obtained U.S. citizenship by marrying a young woman, Helen, who was an American citizen and raised in South Los Angeles. Helen came from a working-class family in the neighborhood where Manuel lived. When Manuel was in his 60s he began to have difficulty with his vision. Because money was tight and he didn't speak English well, he ignored these symptoms. However, over a three-year period his vision became so poor, that Helen urged him to see a doctor. In response to her urging he made an appointment with a physician at a local community health clinic. From there he was referred to an ophthalmologist who diagnosed his vision problems as macular degeneration. The doctor said that he would be blind by age 66. This news devastated Manuel, and over time he developed a habit of staying at home and listening to the radio. Helen maintained her job at a local clothing store and this paid most of their bills. Helen urged Manuel to get out of the house for walks because he stayed home most of the time and had become overweight. At her urging, he did walk around his neighborhood once or twice a week. At 70 years old, Helen urged Manuel, once again, to see a doctor because he was having pain and loss of sensation in his feet and hands. He was diagnosed with late-onset diabetes and was told that unless he could regulate his weight, he would have problems getting around his home and would soon lose function in his hands. Manuel's eye problems precluded him from walking alone, so he became depressed and began drinking alcohol which increased his weight further and exacerbated his diabetic condition.

Manuel's condition is difficult, particularly because some aspects of his situation could have been remedied through a more supportive community environment and with more education. Older adults who have a chronic disability and low income often lack access to health care, which can cause their disability to get worse due to inattention, neglect, and a perceived sense of helplessness to change their situation. In Manuel's case, his wife Helen provided him with some adjunctive support; however, his traditional values, poor English skills, and poverty made it difficult for him to get credible assistance for his disabling condition.

Several studies have documented that an increase in population life expectancy has had the effect of increasing the presence of health problems and disability among older adults (Manton & Saldo, 1992). It has been estimated that 20% of people aged 70 years or older will report a disabling condition that affects activities of daily living, and this percentage increases to 50% in persons aged 85 and older (Alpert, 1994; Ostir et al., 1999; Salive & Guralnik, 1997).

The term *active life expectancy* (ActLE), is useful here as it applies to age-related disability, because it denotes the interaction of disability and age in predicting relative functioning in older adults. Unlike the actuarial term *Active Life Expectancy (ALE)*, ActLE is defined as a gauge of disability that is reflective of the number of years that an older person can expect to live in a condition in which he or she is functional, even in the presence of disability. ActLE is assessed on tasks including instrumental and self-care activities of daily living. (Williams & Temkin-Greener, 1996). One of the implications of ActLE in old age is that as one becomes very old or ages past 85 years it becomes harder to maintain ActLE without assistance. Further, even with assistance, it may not be possible to preserve a full ActLE on some tasks. An example of this phenomenon is captured in the vignette below:

> Alice, age 70, enjoyed working in her garden. At 75 years, she required knee replacement surgery, and although the procedure was successful, her recovery was problematic, and she was only able to kneel down with great difficulty. Returning home, she continued to desire to work in her garden and was fitted with a very low profile rolling walker that allowed her to access limited areas of her garden. However, even with the walker she needed assistance from a live-in aid to engage in gardening activities. Her health deteriorated again when she suffered a stroke at 80 years of age. Her recovery from the stroke left her paralyzed on the left-hand side. It was at this time that she was no longer able to work in her garden, although she continued to pay to have it tended, and enjoyed being walked through the garden in her wheelchair.

This vignette highlights a typical trajectory of loss of ActLE on tasks that have meaning to the individual. Although working in one's garden may not be essential for adaptive living, it represented a source of meaning for Alice. Consequently, developing compensatory strategies that would help Alice stay engaged in the gardening process for as long as possible was an important focus for intervention.

In addition to advanced age, chronic progressive illness is another source of disability and when age and chronic illness interact, this can put an individual at high risk for needing extended assistance to preserve ActLE (Luborsky, 1994). Some of the more persistent chronic illnesses facing adults 70 years and older are listed in Table 8.1, along with their incidence rate in the general population:

TABLE 8.1. PERCENTAGE OF CHRONIC CONDITIONS IN ADULTS
70+ YEARS (U.S. CENTERS FOR DISEASE CONTROL, 1995)

Illness	Female 70+	Male 70+
Stroke	7.9	10.4
Diabetes	11.5	12.9
Cancer	16.7	23.4
Heart Disease	19.2	24.7
Hypertension	48.0	40.5
Arthritis	63.8	49.5

There are a number of factors that influence at what point and to what degree a person will experience disability associated with progressive chronic illness. Several researchers have suggested that construing disability (due to chronic illness) as homogenous oversimplifies its complexity with respect to how it affects ActLE. Verbrugge and Jette (1994) have described disability as a process that produces a gradual erosion of ActLE; however, this model is limited because it doesn't consider individual differences with respect to specific chronic health conditions, nor does it identify specific signs and symptoms that could predict whether a chronic condition would impair functioning to a greater degree in one person versus another. Take for example an older person who has a chronic heart condition. In an ideal situation, this person may receive bypass surgery to correct the condition and with the help of exercise, appropriate medication, and careful lifestyle management have little or no decline in ActLE. In contrast, consider another person with the same heart condition, but who does not receive surgery and as a consequence is homebound because he or she is experiencing chronic fatigue, has pain when walking, and is therefore sedentary. Further, if this second person can't afford medication, the progressive nature of the heart condition could further limit ActLE. In this example, although both persons experience the same chronic heart condition, the impact on ActLE is variable depending on the kinds of resources that are available to deal with the condition and the lifestyle choices of the individual.

Using population-based data from the Women's Health Study (Leveille, Fried, McMullen, & Guralnik, 2004) researchers have identified four areas that could be used to predict whether a disabling condition might impact ActLE. These are: (1) pain, (2) balance impairment, (3) weakness, and (4) diminished endurance. When chronic health conditions are present their impact on reducing ActLE will be greater. Counseling interventions that work to diminish these symptoms will likely be more effective for preserving ActLE in older persons. More research is needed to identify specific features of chronic disease and disability that has the greatest impact on ActLE, however, it is important to note that a future role for counseling is to attend to features of the disabling disease or chronic health condition that are most closely linked to ActLE. A substantial interacting factor in this regard, which is somewhat unique to old age, is when disability is compounded by deterioration in cognitive function.

COGNITIVE IMPAIRMENT AND DISABILITY

Disability due to cognitive impairment deserves special consideration with respect to positive aging, because the nature of well-being and life satisfaction in old age is highly interconnected with the condition of one's mental faculties. The emergence of age-related deteriorative disease states such as Alzheimer's disease (AD) results in an accelerated decline in physical and cognitive functioning and in addition the course of AD is highly progressive with respect to functional loss.

Markers of rapid and profound cognitive deterioration—including deficits in memory, language, abstract thinking, and judgment—are a consequence of AD and shape how an individual ages. An AD sufferer will find it progressively more difficult to maintain functional independence with respect to activities of daily living (ADL) or instrumental activities of daily living (IADL), even if he or she is physically able to perform such tasks.

The potential for cognitive deterioration, disability, and age-related decline to interact in disastrous ways in selected contexts that demand a high degree of mental and physical coordination are underscored in a *New York Times* report (LeDuff, 2003) of an 87-year-old man who drove his car into pedestrians at a farmer's market in Santa Monica, CA. The incident had disastrous consequences, including the deaths of 10 people. One of the reasons offered to explain this accident, was the possibility that the older driver was experiencing cognitive problems that impaired his ability to drive his car safely.

Driving is one of the most complex everyday living skills that older adults must negotiate, involving not only memory and attention skills, but substantial eye, foot, and hand coordination. To drive adequately requires quick reaction time across changing dynamic contexts, along with a significant degree of spatial problem solving. Nothing about driving a car happens slowly. Every driver must be able to stop, go, turn left, right, respond to noises (horns honking), discriminate between sounds (radio versus a ambulance siren), retrieve information in the form of traffic rules and regulations, and apply them, sometimes instantaneously, during a changing dynamic context (when to switch lanes, when and how to turn left, when to yield, etc.). On the other hand, driving is a prized source of independence for Americans. Almost every activity of daily living in many places in America depends on the ability to drive. So, losing one's driving privilege can have negative repercussions not only for a sense of well-being, but also for addressing the instrumental realities of everyday living such as shopping for groceries.

In a longitudinal study that was undertaken to evaluate the impact of Alzheimer's disease on driving performance, researchers at Washington University in St. Louis, Missouri, administered a performance road test every six months to a sample of 108 older adults, 58 of whom were not cognitively impaired, 21 who had very mild cognitive impairment due to AD, and 29 who had mild to moderate AD (Duchek et al., 2003). At baseline, all participants were able to pass the driving test, which consisted of a range of typical behaviors that would be required for competent driving, such as signaling and changing lanes, stopping at stop signs, parking, and distinguishing between the brake and the gas pedal. The goal of this study was to determine if the rate of failure over time on this performance test increased as a function of disease severity. As expected, those with more severe AD failed the driving test sooner and at a higher rate than either the mildly impaired or unimpaired groups. The researchers concluded that cognitive problems such as those found in AD put a person at serious risk for making major driver errors. AD, therefore, is a disease of cognitive function that represents a serious disablement risk factor for driving.

In this case disability would be defined as the loss of one's capacity to drive an automobile. Losing the ability to drive a car independently due to age/disease-related cognitive deterioration is not a discrete event; rather, it involves a process of age-related decline that moves toward a threshold point of safe versus not safe driving. For this reason, a positive aging approach to driving in old age would involve managing one's capacities in relation to the skills needed to safely drive in the presence of age-related decline.

With respect to positive aging, it is not only important to identify when cognitive problems become severe enough to impact functioning, but it is also important to suggest strategies for addressing such deficits so a person can remain functionally independent for as long as possible. From the *New York Times* report cited above, identifying the point that a person can no longer drive a car independently was a critical issue and the failure to do so had disastrous consequences for not only the pedestrians, but for the older driver as well. However, factors that motivated this older person to get in his car and drive should also be understood with respect to a person's inherent need to preserve his or her ActLE for as long as possible, and to use the routines that he or she has developed over a lifetime to accomplish this. Would it have been possible, in this case, for the elderly man to meet his functional needs without having to drive?

This question raises important concerns for interventions that attempt to preserve ActLE in persons with cognitive impairment who are at risk for driving problems. Accurate assessment is essential in people with cognitive impairment. Chapter 4 reviewed general functional assessment tools used to identify cognitive problems in older people. Although such instruments can be helpful in flagging whether a disease process is present to assess whether a person is able to drive an automobile or operate complex household equipment (dishwasher, oven) that requires not only physical dexterity but also cognitive capacity, involves a somewhat different approach.

A recent review of studies that examined automobile driving in an older person with suspected cognitive problems provided some useful guidelines for geriatric practitioners. Alternatives to what appeared to be the most important way to assess this skill was to actually test the person's ability to drive (Brown & Ott, 2004). This would mean a realistic test of driving and observing of errors. If this is not possible, other strategies might be to ask specific questions of caregivers or loved ones that pinpoint driving errors. Questions would include whether the passenger observes an older driver getting lost, running stop signs, staying on the road, finding the controls to change a side mirror, going too fast or too slow in relationship to the posted speed limit, and inability to park easily. This level of specificity can be an indicator of whether a person should continue to drive (Taylor & Tripodes, 2001).

Perhaps the best test is to simply drive with the person, directly observing his or her driving skills. Even in this case, observation may create an artificial testing environment that does not match real-world activity. If driving is no longer possible, a positive aging intervention that aims at preserving the older person's dignity as well as his or her ActLE is critical. The National Alzheimer's Association has provided recommendations to follow should the decision be made to revoke a person's privilege to drive. This listing includes: (1) have the person take a driving test and acknowledge the loss of driving skill and ability; (2) arrange for other options for transportation as a way to preserve ActLE; (3) encourage support from others in the person's social context such as family, friends, and neighbors; (4) remove the car so that it does not remind the person of a lost privilege; (5) do not send mixed messages by returning driving privileges (National Alzheimer's Association, 1995).

Management of persons with cognitive problems, with the goal of preserving ActLE, is challenging, and research is needed to develop intervention approaches that help such persons acknowledge this issue and its impact on functional independence. Several important management processes are critical in this regard including monitoring the client, limiting activities that are impacted by the cognitive deficit, helping the patient acknowledge and be receptive of help from caregivers or professionals, and finding alternative ways for the client to get his or her everyday living needs met.

CAREGIVING

Informal caregiving, in its most elemental form characterizes a family member, loved one, neighbor, or significant other who provides direct assistance to a person (a care recipient) who, due to disability, is in need of assistance. Caregiving involves help with activities necessary to function independently at home or in the community and, in more severe cases, extends to instrumental help with self-care behaviors including bathing, eating, dressing, and grooming. It is a pervasive activity that occurs across the United States and there are many persons who have been caregivers or been confronted with this issue in extended relationships. In a telephone survey commissioned in 2001 by AARP of 4037 adults surveyed, 34% reported that they had been involved in caregiving (AARP, 2001). Extrapolating from this telephone survey suggests that nearly 65 million persons have been (or are currently) caregivers. Not surprisingly, the majority of those who reported that they were caregivers were over 50 years of age.

The caregiving task is influenced by a number of factors related to the specific needs of the care recipient. Physical impairment might include osteoarthritis, osteoporosis, severe muscle weakness, profound sensory deficits, or disability due to a disease condition such as cardiovascular disease or cancer. Cognitive impairment includes persons suffering from Alzheimer's disease or other forms of dementia, and cognitive deficits due to stroke. Caregiving may be more or less challenging given the type and severity of a person's cognitive or physical disability. For individuals who are cognitively intact, but are not physically able, there is potential for meaningful social communication as part of the caregiving activity. This may not be the case when the care recipient has a degenerative brain disease such as AD. Understanding the nature and cause of the care recipient's disability and its effects on the caregiver are important in a positive aging approach to caregiving.

A prominent stereotype of caregiving is that it is a burdensome task with only negative consequences for the caregiver, including depression, anxiety, poor health, and hopelessness. Interestingly, the research literature underscores a more complex scenario that is related to the: (1) care recipient's problems or difficulties; (2) the physical and psychological resources of the caregiver; and (3) the relationship between the caregiver and the care recipient. From a positive aging perspective, it is important that this array of factors is acknowledged in order to understand the inherent benefits and challenges of caregiving. The literature is replete with the negative aspects of caregiving and several studies have highlighted these (George & Gwyther, 1986; Schulz, O'Brien, Bookwala, & Fleissner, 1995; Tennstedt, Cafferata, & Sullivan, 1992). The specific challenges of caregiving are captured in the Caregiver Burden Scale (Bedard et al., 2001) including: personal time lost to caregiving, the stress of multiple demands, anger and resentment toward the care recipient, personal health problems of the caregiver that make the provision of care more challenging, loss of privacy, diminishment of one's social network, loss of personal control, uncertainty about the future, and feelings of inadequacy around providing care.

Of importance in a positive aging perspective on caregiving is not only an awareness of its challenges, but the acknowledgment that caring for a loved one who is physically or cognitively disabled due to age-related deterioration can be a source of positive consequences as well. The positive benefits that emerge from a caregiving relationship are related to opportunities associated with helping a loved one in need. In some cases, such an altruistic orientation has been conceptualized as a buffer for the stress of providing care (Broerner, Schulz, & Horowitz, 2004). Several features of the caregiving context have been examined as sources of positive emotions toward caregiving, including the seriousness of the care recipient's disability and whether the care recipient can communicate clearly what help is needed. In addition, if a care recipient is cognitively intact then he or she might express appreciation for help received. Another source of positive aging can be found in the ongoing relationship between the caregiver and the care recipient (Barusch & Spaid, 1996). A caregiver who has been in a long-term marriage or relationship with a care recipient, which has been a source of positive personal meaning, may welcome the opportunity to care for a deteriorating partner as a way of increasing the meaningfulness of the relationship. If, on the other hand, the relationship between caregiver and care recipient has been problematic in the past, then caregiving may become an additional source of strain on the relationship (Barusch & Spaid, 1996). Given this latter scenario, it may be useful for the caregiver and care recipient to seek out professional counseling to help them resolve differences in their relationship. Working toward resolving relationship difficulty could ease some of the burdens associated with care (Gallagher-Thompson, Dal Canto, Jacob, & Thompson, 2001).

In one longitudinal study (Beach, Schulz, Yee, & Jackson, 2000) of 680 respondents from the Cardiovascular Health Study (CHS; Fried et al., 1991), approximately half of whom identified themselves as caregivers, there was a sense of improved mental health in those persons who were providing care. Among the various findings from this study was that caring for a spouse who was in the early stages of disability was associated with decreased psychological symptoms and a positive attitude toward helping. While it should be noted that this study was confined to care recipients whose primary problems were physical disability, the findings highlight the point that the act of helping can have positive consequences for a caregiver.

A positive aging approach to caregiving might emphasize both the challenges and perceived benefits of caregiving. Most caregiver burden scales exclusively focus on the difficulties that a caregiver encounters in such relationships. Future research might also examine sources of positive strength and resources that emerge from the caregiving relationship. The positive aspects of caregiving should, of course, be balanced with the kinds of problems that a caregiver encounters and the skill and psychological resources of the caregiver. When problems become severe, such as in more advanced stages of AD or when severe physical disability creates substantial self-care issues, such as incontinence or sleep disruption, then it may be that professional help is needed. However, even in these more difficult cases, finding ways for a caregiver to be involved in the care of a loved one who has been a source of positive meaning for a person over the life span may be important to consider in the development of interventions and strategies designed to optimize caregiving and promote positive aging.

Extended Care Environments

When an older person can no longer live at home or cannot live independently, even with the assistance of an informal or professional live-in caregiver, then extended care is needed outside the home. The use of extended care as a way to maintain positive aging should involve an approach that helps the older disabled adult maintain a sense of dignity and even some degree of self-sufficiency by emphasizing social and environmental continuity.

SOC provides information that could inform the nature and design of extended residential care with respect to how such care contexts could be designed to promote positive aging in disabled older adults. From within the framework of SOC, such care could be considered a form of selectivity inasmuch as the primary function of extended care is to remove the individual from the community. It also is the case that extended care involves optimization and compensation by creating an artificial living context where fewer demands are placed on the individual. For example, prepared meals and even assistance eating are common in residential care facilities, balanced by allowing the resident to make choices of food type and level of feeding assistance needed. This is done because, for a substantially impaired older person, even a few demands can quickly overwhelm the individual and thereby magnify the effects of the impairment. However, even in the presence of profound disability, opportunities for making decisions and choices, even though these are restricted in such a living environment are essential to emotional well-being. Therefore, involving the older resident (and the family) in determining how restrictive the environment should become is important in optimizing care.

With increased disability there is a high degree of need to optimize the skills and capabilities that remain intact within the individual, while at the same time compensating for lost skills (e.g., balancing optimization and compensation).

Jackie was admitted to a residential care facility because her family was no longer able to care for her due to progressive Alzheimer's disease. An assessment of Jackie's cognitive functioning placed her in the moderate range of dementia. She had a fairly high level of anxiety and agitation at times. Jackie was unable to orient herself to person, place, and time; however, she had a fairly good memory for autobiographical material and particularly for playing piano tunes that she had learned earlier in life. Interestingly, although Jackie had substantial memory loss, her piano playing skill was, for the most part, preserved, particularly on highly overlearned pieces of music. Jackie was admitted to the care unit and was encouraged by the staff to become involved in a number of activities. Her family indicated that she enjoyed playing the piano, so she was allowed supervised access to it and her playing was taped. She was encouraged to play only simple tunes that she remembered and had overlearned (selection), and this became a source of entertainment to the residents as she replayed and practiced familiar tunes (optimization). As she became progressively more demented, her piano skills worsened. In this instance she

189

continued to sit at the piano bench listening to the tapes of songs she had played in the past (compensation). The residents enjoyed this taped music as well, and it brought satisfaction to Jackie because even though she no longer actually played the pieces, the residents still attributed the taped music to her piano playing. These strategies also helped to manage her anxiety and agitation without medication. This was likely due to the fact that piano playing involved her in a familiar and comforting activity, thus preserving her sense of continuity.

By conceptualizing resident behaviors in terms of selection, optimization, and compensation, it is possible to develop individualized treatment plans designed to maximize resident functioning, even in the presence of declining capacity. Aspects of the SOC model have been adopted in some of the more progressive extended care strategies. Two important themes for maintaining positive aging in the presence of age-related functional decline in extended care environments are: (1) aging in place and (2) matching stages of decline with levels of care.

The term *aging in place*, refers to both a philosophy and a practice of providing health and personal care services to older people in the least restrictive and most homelike setting possible, even as those people become increasingly ill and impaired. The important part of the aging in place concept is that as people age, they retain the need for a living environment in which they feel their identity and autonomy are preserved. Older people who retain all or nearly all of their functional capacity are able to remain in their own homes or choose one of a variety of living environments. However, a living environment that proactively assists the preservation of autonomy, even when physical or cognitive decline becomes prominent, would represent a model of aging in place.

An important consideration in creating an extended care environment that can address the deteriorative and progressive nature of age-related disability is matching the level of care provided with the stages of decline of the individual. *Stages of decline* is a concept useful in the process of making such choices with respect to care needs. Figure 8.1 provides a graphic representation of how the stages of decline relate to levels of care (Thorn 2002).

When disability is relatively minimal, the need for care will be minor. Very little assistance is likely to be needed to help the person

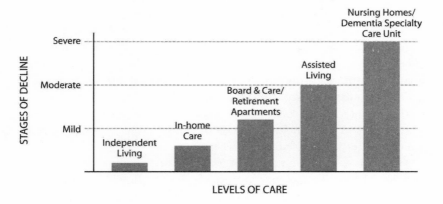

FIGURE 8.1. Stages of decline and care needs (Thorn, 2002, p. 30).

maintain quality of life and well-being with respect to independence and self-sufficiency. As the disability progresses, more extended kinds of care are needed; that is, in order for a person to maintain a sense of well-being, a higher level of care is required. If level of care and stages of decline are not matched, the process can be a barrier to positive aging. When older adults who are living independently (low need) contemplate a future in a nursing home when they become old (level of care is unknown), a negative reaction is predictable. In one large study of hospitalized elderly patients, 56% of respondents stated that they would be "very unwilling" to enter a nursing home or would "rather die" than be placed against their will in a nursing home care facility (Mattimore et al. 1997). It is stressful, discouraging, and often painful to suffer the illness or chronic health problems that could trigger the placement of an older person in a long-term care facility. The dread of spending time in a context where the level of care is far greater than the stage of perceived decline, however, can lead to a sense of powerlessness and apathy.

The Eden Alternative™

The Eden Alternative™ is an innovative approach to extended care environments that incorporates aging-in-place concepts. It was first proposed by William Thomas, MD, in the early 1990s. As a physician-director of a nursing home, Dr. Thomas rethought a number of institutional problems inherent in the medical model underlying nursing home care. The most important feature of his Eden Alternative model was the idea that the home environment epitomizes the nature of care that is most acceptable to human beings. Thus, the incorporation of homelike facilities, including mechanisms to bring children into the facility, are encouraged. Further, animals, birds, and plants are planned aspects of the environment so that typically, one might find domesticated birds and a variety of pets including dogs and cats present in any given Eden Alternative facility. Judy Thomas, a partner in the Eden Alternative, was quoted in a *Washington Post* article as saying that Eden Alternative facilities are designed to be flexible and reflect, as closely as possible, the routines, schedules, and lifestyle patterns that are found at home (Levine, 1997).

The Eden Alternative represents one effort to engender an institutionalized model of long-term care that emphasizes principles of positive aging by designing a care context that attempts to match level of care and stage of decline by allowing resident choice for as long as possible through a supportive physical structure that emphasizes connectedness among residents and the professional staff. This philosophy emulates an ideal family-based context where caregivers and care recipients are in an ongoing interdependent living context. Aspects of the Eden Alternative model that make it consistent with a positive aging approach to residential care include: (1) understanding that loneliness and helplessness account for the majority of problems in long-term care; (2) development of a place that emphasizes the residents' humanity; (3) easy access to companionship; (4) opportunities to give and receive care; (5) deemphasis of top-down bureaucratic authority; (6) leadership that focuses on the need to improve resident quality of life over institutionalization concerns; (7) an approach to care that attempts to match the level (or intensity of care) with the specific stage of decline of each individual resident.

There is currently an absence of empirical data that can provide information as to whether this specific model of extended care is more effective than other models of residential care facilities such as board and care. In these informal extended care settings, a private home is literally converted to an assisted living environment (see Hill & Gregg, 2002); however, the flexibility to deal with the wide range of impaired older adults, particularly, those who need 24-hour nursing care, is limited in board and care facilities (Thorn, 2002). Further, it is not known whether such home-care strategies can meaningfully address the great variation of needs as residents become more impaired cognitively and behaviorally. However, conceptually, home-based alternatives represent innovative approaches to care that are consistent with the notion of positive aging.

CONCLUDING COMMENTS

This chapter examined disability in old age and how it affects the aging process. A positive aging approach for dealing with disability was described, including the concept of active life expectancy (ActLE) and how this term is related to a positive aging framework for addressing age-related disability. Cognitive impairment, as a special form of disability, was examined. Issues of caregiving were explored and a positive aging strategy for optimizing quality of life and well-being in caregiving was suggested. The role of extended care environments, including a framework for gauging disability in terms of balancing impairment with "levels of care," was described. The Eden Alternative was described as an example of a positive aging approach to long-term care.

Chapter 9

POSITIVE AGING IN GRIEF,
BEREAVEMENT, DEATH,
AND DYING

FOR LONG-TERM MARRIED couples or those in a long-term dyadic relationship, it is inevitable that at some point during the course of the relationship, most commonly in old age, one partner will succumb to death before the other. This is an embedded part of our social fabric, and for this reason social and cultural traditions have evolved in ways that have acknowledged this reality. Western, Judeo-Christian matrimonial vows, for example, often include the phrase, "until death do us part." However, even though the loss of a spouse or long-term partner to death is inevitable, and that loss is likely to occur among persons who are older, such a loss is one of the more emotionally difficult challenges that an older person can face (Gallagher, Breckenridge, Thompson, & Peterson, 1983).

The loss of a family member or loved one has been characterized in a number of ways; however, the research literature has identified primarily two terms that capture its emotional consequences and social phenomenology; namely, grief and bereavement. Grief is the psychological or intrapersonal experience of loss while bereavement describes the process that a person engages to deal with loss. It is during the bereavement process that grieving occurs, and a surviving spouse is recognized as a widow or widower and given permission to mourn the loss. The scientific literature that examines grief and bereavement in old age focuses, for the most part, on spousal loss, and for this reason, it is useful to summarize some of this research to lay the groundwork for discussing positive aging as a source of adaptation and coping with grief and bereavement in old age.

The incidence of spousal loss to death has been estimated to occur in the United States among the elderly at 1.6% yearly for men and over 3% yearly for women (Murrell, Norris, & Hutchings, 1984). More contemporary demographic projections have estimated that for persons 70 years of age and older, as many as 60% of women and 14% of men will report having been widowed at some point during their lifetime (Sadock & Sadock, 2003). The fact that conjugal loss occurs at roughly three times the rate in old age as it does in youth or middle adulthood (U.S. Census, 1997) makes it predominantly an older adult concern.

The research on stress and human functioning considers the loss of a spouse to death at any point across the life span to be one of the most challenging events that a person can experience (Holmes & Rahe, 1967). And, not surprisingly, a predictable reaction to the loss of a spouse is distress, including acute psychopathology such as depression or anxiety (Gallagher et al., 1983). Although most surviving spouses recover from such a loss, a sizable percentage of persons remain vulnerable or at risk for chronic emotional illness. Early in the bereavement process, research has documented that there is nearly a 50% chance that a surviving spouse will report symptoms of depression, including hopelessness, sleep disturbance, low energy, and profound sadness (Thompson, Breckenridge, Gallagher, & Peterson, 1984; Clayton, 1979; Harlow, Goldberg, & Comstock, 1991). Epidemiological studies have reported that as high as 25% of widows may continue to experience the symptoms of clinical depression even after a year of grieving (Zisook & Shuchter, 1986). In addition to depression, older widows and widowers may experience symptoms of anxiety as well (Schut, de Keijser, van den Bout, & Dijkhuis, 1991). These statistics underscore the substantial emotional upheaval that occurs during grieving.

There may also be negative health consequences for a surviving spouse, particularly if the survivor was in poor mental or physical health prior to the loss. Although declines in physical health associated with the grieving and bereavement process would seem intuitive, data in support of this contention are somewhat mixed (Murrell, Meeks, & Walker, 1991); however, the majority of evidence suggests that recent widow(ers), particularly within a year of spousal loss, will frequently feel sick or ill-at-ease, and they may self-report more physical symptoms than similar aged persons who are married (Fenwick & Barresi, 1981). There is also evidence that newly widowed older adults tend to take more medications, visit their doctor more often, and complain more frequently of stress and fatigue than persons of similar age who are not grieving (Osterweis, Solomon, & Green, 1984).

From the point of view of continuity theory, the loss of a spouse to death represents a substantial discontinuity, particularly if the preloss relationship was happy and a source of emotional support for the surviving partner. Older widow(ers) on average, experience lower levels of distress than younger widows (Stroebe & Stroebe, 1993) and this may be explained by a number of reasons: (1) In old age there is the recognition that life is approaching an end and partner loss is a late-life inevitability. (2) In one's older years it is often the case that a fixed retirement income continues after the partner's death, so the survivor does not lose socioeconomically due to the loss. (3) Children are grown and there are few, if any, ongoing childrearing demands. In fact, it may be the case that adult children play a role in helping their surviving parent cope with the loss.

Because the degree of discontinuity of widowhood is lower in later life than in youth, there is an opportunity to develop compensation strategies to deal with conjugal loss in old age. The literature that has examined the psychological aspects of coping with spousal loss has focused on what are called "protective factors" as these are associated with recovery from the distress associated with grieving (Stroebe & Stroebe, 1993).

PROTECTIVE FACTORS IN GRIEF AND BEREAVEMENT

Researchers have defined protective factors as specific resources available to the surviving spouse that work to buffer the stress of mourning (Murrell et al., 1991). Two that characterize positive aging are: (1) social support and (2) regulating one's emotional responsivity.

Social support has been studied as a protective factor for the grieving spouse given that in old age, widow(ers) are often part of an immediate family that includes children and in-laws, and are often connected to an extended family network that includes siblings and more distant kin. If an older widow(er) is part of a supportive social network, it is likely that people in this network will have a vested interest in supporting the grieving spouse as a way to maintain continuity of the social support system. For children of the surviving spouse, it may be that their availability to the grieving parent is a way to help them deal with their own sense of grief surrounding the loss of their parent (Abeles, Victor, & Delano-Wood, 2004). It is not surprising, therefore, that many older widow(ers) turn to immediate and extended family members for understanding and sympathy, particularly during the early stages of the bereavement process. In several studies the presence of social support, particularly if it is sensitive to the needs of the surviving spouse, has been found to be helpful in reestablishing a sense of well-being and life satisfaction during the course of bereavement (Stroebe, Stroebe, Abakoumkin, & Schut, 1996; Worden, 1991).

A critical aspect of the provision of social support is whether it is perceived by the grieving spouse as meaningful and helpful (Norris & Murrell, 1990). Meaningful social support embodies specific behaviors including empathic listening, encouraging the mourner to find meaning in the present, the provision of instrumental help including meals, assistance in transitioning possessions of the deceased spouse, and helping the mourner shift his or her identity from that of a married to a single person (Rando, 1998). Interestingly, the presence of others in one's social network who could potentially be helpful, but who fail to follow through and provide instrumental assistance could make coping even more difficult; therefore, what people actually do or the behaviors they engage in to assist the older grieving spouse is perhaps more important than just being available to help him or her.

Interestingly, even when the surviving spouse is receiving support, some recently widowed persons may feel that supportive help from others is inadequate (Bankoff, 1983). Therefore, a critical aspect in understanding how social support can alleviate suffering is the assessment of functional (or instrumental) components of social support. In some instances, the quality of the support provided may be poor; for example, if the support system is out of sync with the surviving spouse's recovery needs (Davidowitz & Myrick, 1984). In some instances others in the grieving person's social support system may grow tired or impatient with the grieving process. When this happens a grieving spouse may feel pressure to cease grieving and "get on with life." If a surviving spouse is not emotionally ready to move on, this kind of premature prodding can create more discouragement and despondency (Lehman, Ellard, & Wortman, 1986; Wortman & Lehman, 1985). Therefore, although social support is generally construed as a protective factor for persons grieving the loss of a loved one, the subjective nature of the support is important to maximize the effectiveness of social support as a positive aging resource for coping.

Emotional regulation is another factor that has been found to influence bereavement loss. A common stereotype of the grieving process is that it involves substantial distress, psychic pain, and suffering that must take place in order for the widow(er) to fully reconcile him- or herself with the loss. However, some research has suggested that the ability to generate positive emotions during the grieving process may buffer the stress associated with bereavement (Ong, Bergeman, & Bisconti, 2004). Although it is somewhat antithetical to consider positive emotions as a source of relief from the work of grieving, the clinical and research literature has highlighted a number of specific emotional states, such as humor, that have been found to moderate the intensity of the grief response. For example, Bonanno (1999) has pointed out that common traditions of storytelling about the life of the deceased, including reminiscing about humorous moments in the departed person's life, can have the effect of breaking the cycle of pain and suffering associated with grieving. The ability to cultivate positive emotional states may be one intrapersonal resource that characterizes resilient coping in widowhood.

The potential to experience a range of emotional responses to the grief and mourning process can also be seen in the cultural or traditional variations that different subgroups within our Western culture deal with the death of loved ones. As an example, the Mexican-American custom of Dia de los Muertos (the Day of the Dead) highlights the interrelationship between festiveness and sadness as a way to help members of this cultural group reconcile themselves to the feelings of loss when a loved one dies. An excerpt from John West's book, *Mexican Folklore* (1988) summarizes this custom:

> Families with Mexican roots [take] with them rakes and hoes and water buckets, along with picnic lunches [to the family grave sites]. Prominent also are mounds of flowers in every color imaginable. . . . Graves have their weeds cut; mounds are remolded and sprinkled with water. Names on wooden crosses . . . are straightened up . . . Then the family, seated around the grave, has a picnic meal . . . for it is truly a family gathering, a [symbolic] visit with members of the family who have "gone ahead." (p. 152)

The Role of the Professional Counselor

Grief counseling to assist the bereaved is a ubiquitous term that captures a wide range of intervention approaches from standard psychotherapy such as cognitive behavioral therapy (Fleming & Robinson, 2001; Hill, Packard, & Lund, 1996) to more existential intervention strategies such as life review (Butler, 1963). A common theme across grief counseling approaches is to encourage the surviving loved one to come to terms with new self-perceptions (i.e., from being married to becoming a single adult), and to engage in activities that have the potential to restore the sense of preloss wellbeing or happiness. Embedded in these approaches is the idea that it is possible to recover from the loss of a spouse by proactively coping with its emotional consequences.

This process, was captured in the findings from the Changing Lives of Older Couples study (CLOC; Bonanno, Wortman, & Nesse, 2004), which surveyed a group of 185 older persons who lived in the Detroit–Chicago area and who had recently lost a spouse to death. These participants were drawn from a larger group of 1532 married persons of whom this subgroup of participants had experienced the loss of their spouse to death during the course of the study. A powerful feature of the CLOC study was the assessment of these 185 CLOC participants before and after the loss. Specifically, the surviving spouse was assessed by virtue of the longitudinal study design several years before the loss (the preloss phase) and at approximately 6 and 18 months following the loss (postloss phase).

199

Interestingly, although most of these CLOC widow(ers) reported distress and trauma near the time of the death of their spouse, over 50% indicated (at the 6-month follow-up) that they were experiencing little or no distress and hardly any grief.

The researchers labeled these individuals "resilient respondents." Several features of resilient respondents are worth noting. First, they engaged in active coping; namely, they worked hard to generate positive emotions including cultivating and rehearsing good memories about their deceased spouse. Second, they became active in purposeful life pursuits which helped them develop new lifestyle patterns and behaviors. In addition to resilient responders, Bonanno and his colleagues identified a small group of participants who comprised about 10% of their sample and whom they labeled "depressed-improved" respondents. These were persons whose marriage (preloss) was perceived as poor or problematic for various reasons. For example, a few were caregivers of a cognitively impaired partner. This depressed-improved group evidenced even better emotional health after the death of their partner than they reported while their partner was alive.

There were also several groups of respondents who continued to experience grief or depression for as long as 18 months postloss. These were labeled the "chronic grief" and the "chronic depression" respondents. Chronic grievers self-reported substantial distress around the loss and this created a persistent form of disequilibrium. They believed for various reasons, that they could not continue without their lost partner. These respondents tended to dwell on the loss event and the trauma associated with the dying process of the spouse. The chronic depression respondents, on the other hand, reported a life-span history of psychopathology including clinical depression. Their symptoms were exacerbated by the loss. In these latter two groups, the level and persistence of self-reported grief probably warranted professional counseling.

One implication of the findings from the CLOC study for the practicing grief counselor is the importance of assessing the nature of the preloss relationship or marriage. In addition it is also important to know how the grieving client was functioning emotionally before his or her partner died. In Chapter 4, several instruments were described to measure emotional functioning in old age including the Geriatric Depression Scale and an anxiety screening tool to assess for the presence of depressed or anxious affect. These instruments may be useful in assessing a bereaving person's current emotional state although they were not designed specifically for bereavement.

There are, however, a number of instruments that are tailored to grief, including the Bereavement Response Scale II (Weiss & Richards, 1997) and the Grief Measurement Scale (Jacobs, Kasl, & Ostfeld, 1986). The Texas Revised Inventory of Grief (Faschingbauer, Zisook, & DeVaul, 1987) is a measure that was developed to assess multiple aspects of the grieving process including intensity of grieving in the past (e.g., "I found it hard to work well after this person died") and the impact of grieving in the present (e.g., "I still cry when I think of the person who died"). Using this instrument, the grief counselor can gauge not only the older grieving client's current emotional state, but also the degree to which the client is able to grieve over time. This scale can be purchased from American Psychiatric Press and is one assessment tool that the grief counselor might employ in intervention planning. The Grief Resolution Index, available from Remondet and Hansson (1987) measures whether the person has reconciled him- or herself to a partner's death. This index consists of seven items summarized as follows: (1) accepted the death of my [partner]; (2) stopped saying "we"; (3) became able to reach out to others; (4) able to do my crying and get it over with; (5) said goodbye to my [partner]; (6) able to think through what my [partner's] death meant to me; (7) able to get on with my new life. The client rates each of these items on a 5-point scale that measures functioning with respect to each of the seven items (from 1 = very poorly to 5 = very well). This instrument could identify areas where a widow or widower may be experiencing problems in regaining a sense of well-being and may also be helpful in determining whether a person may be able to manage his or her emotions in the recovery process.

The findings from the CLOC study suggest that positive aging can be found in a person's ability to reframe challenges in a more positive light and to actively regulate his or her emotions, even in the face of difficulty. Engaging positive emotional states can counter negative thinking and facilitate recovery from the distress associated with grief. In a study that tested the impact of positive emotion on coping and bereavement in later life, Ong and Colleagues (Ong et al., 2004) assessed approximately 30 elderly widow(ers) a few days after the death of their spouse. They found that those widow(ers) who were able to generate positive emotions during grieving, such as humor or the generation of a positive perspective, were better able to cope with the loss. This was in contrast to those who tended to focus on negative emotions who then had more difficulty letting go of grief. In short, those widow(ers) who were better at generating positive emotions fared better emotionally and were protected from psychopathology. These researchers also concluded that interventions focusing on activities that cultivate positive emotions and a sense of personal self-improvement (such as physical exercise as a way to take one's mind off grieving) would be the most helpful in facilitating recovery from grief-related distress.

Chapter 7 highlighted several meaning-based life-span strategies that could be employed as part of a positive aging counseling intervention designed to generate positive emotions and rally meaningful social support. One method for challenging persistent negative behaviors might be to begin a gratitude journal in which one records opportunities to be grateful for living as a way to find positive meaning in life (Emmons & McCullough, 2003). A more behaviorally oriented meaning-based strategy might be volunteer work (Morrow-Howell et al., 2003). If such "other-oriented" behavior engages the widow(er) in directly helping others the process may help the bereaved spouse find new sources of meaning. During the early stages of bereavement, research points to the value of support groups or engaging with other persons who are also working through the bereavement process (Lehman et al., 1986). In terms of social support, if those who are offering help or assistance to the grieving person engage in active listening and the provision of opportunities for the grieving spouse to express his or her feelings about the loss (while at the same time encouraging the rehearsal of positive memories) recovery is likely. Shaping of responses that focus on the positive aspects of the preloss relationship and the memories that this relationship engendered should be beneficial with respect to grief recovery. The case study that follows highlights a grief counseling approach that incorporates a positive aging perspective.

Helen is 73 years old. She and her husband Mark had been married for 50 years until Mark's death the previous year from lung cancer. Helen and Mark were happily married and they had four children from their union. They also had several grandchildren. The circumstances around Mark's death were related to his long-term cigarette smoking habit and his inability to quit smoking, even after he was diagnosed with lung cancer. Although Helen reported that her marriage was happy, she also reported intermittent periods of time when she suffered from clinical depression. During these episodes, Mark was very supportive of Helen's situation and was instrumental in helping her recover her emotional well-being. In this regard, Helen was highly dependent on Mark for emotional stability. Although Mark's death was not a surprise because it followed after a year of very poor health, it precipitated a recurrence of Helen's clinical depression. After six months of unrelenting grief Helen made an appointment with her therapist, who was familiar with Helen's history. The therapist assessed Helen's situation and discovered that a number of symptoms that were similar to her previous depressive episodes were present. The therapist encouraged Helen to see a psychiatrist who restarted her antidepressant medication. The psychiatrist also prescribed benzodiazepines to help her control her anxiety. The therapist then engaged Helen in individual psychotherapy to help her develop strategies for finding meaning in her life in the absence of Mark. Helen decided to return to activity in her local church and it was there that she reconnected with some old friends. Two of her children attended the same church and this increased their interaction with Helen. The therapist also suggested that Helen begin a project that she wanted to start for herself but was previously too busy to begin. After some time, she decided to write her personal history, and as part of that process, trace her genealogical records back four generations. Part of this project involved visits to the library and local records department. The therapist met weekly with Helen and monitored her depressive symptoms, medication, and her social relationships. During the course of therapy he also suggested that Helen begin a gratitude journal, writing about events and activities in the present and future that she was grateful for. She did this on a daily basis for several weeks and found that it lifted her mood. Slowly, Helen began to report feeling somewhat better. Signs that she was transitioning out of her chronic grieving were noticeable, including her tendency with the passage of time to speak less and less about Mark.

There is a growing literature that highlights specific intervention approaches like the one described above that operate from a positive aging perspective (Rando, 1998; Worden, 1991). In general, this literature suggests that effective interventions for older adults caught in sustained bereavement should: (1) assess the nature of the preloss relationship as well as the nature of grieving in the past and in the present; (2) help the client frame the loss with respect to developing new meaning for living without the partner; (3) assist the client in regulating his or her emotional response to the loss and, over time, encourage the cultivation of positive emotions which should help the client find resources for well-being and satisfaction in life (Bonanno & Kaltman, 1999).

POSITIVE AGING IN DEATH AND DYING

The adage that "no one lives forever" underscores the interpretation that dying is an inevitable outcome in old and very old age (Bradley, Fried, Kasl, & Idler, 2000). Erickson's final stage of life-span development, summarized in Chapter 2, highlights the dying process as the ultimate task in acquiring positive maturational characteristics in old age including "Wisdom vs. Despair." Given that dying is the final milestone for cultivating a positive aging approach to living and, because dying is often associated with pain and suffering, the clinical and scientific literature has suggested that for some older persons, contemplating one's own dying can be associated with a host of negative emotional states (Niemeyer, 1988; Tomer & Eliason, 1996). On the other hand the act of dying in old age, given that the person is cognitively intact, can result in a feeling of closure around a life well-lived. A framework for understanding death and dying from a normal developmental perspective is presented with respect to theories that characterize the dying process as it occurs in old age. Positive aging and its connection to dying is then described from within this theoretical context using principles that are most likely to promote a positive emotional response to the dying process.

The process of dying has been described in a number of ways and there is debate as to whether dying is best captured as a state, a series of stages, or a trajectory (George, 2002). However, all theories of dying converge around the idea that death is a process with some predictable patterns that involve transitioning emotional and physical states (Copp, 1998). The two theories of dying described next focus on different aspects of this phenomenon. The first describes stages that a person may experience as he or she nears death. The second characterizes death and the process of dying as a psychological state with an anticipatory attitude about the event. This latter approach also suggests that one's psychological state changes over time as life's end nears. This viewpoint of dying is of particular interest because it opens the door to intervention approaches designed to alter one's psychological state and that may have application in assisting an older person who is negotiating the dying process. Both of these theories of dying are useful in laying the foundation for a positive aging approach to dying as well as the role of the professional counselor as a facilitator of positive aging and well-being during the dying process.

Dying was characterized early on by researchers in the field of gerontology as a process that involves a series of discrete stages that a person negotiates as he or she nears the end of life. The nature of these stages and whether one moves through them sequentially or cycles back to earlier stages is difficult to know. However, Kübler-Ross's (1969) initial conceptualization of the stages of dying suggested that a person needed to work through each stage in order for quality of life to be preserved during the dying process. Kübler-Ross conceptualized her approach to the dying process based on extensive experience with over 200 dying patients (across all ages) with whom she had professional contact. Dying, in her view occurs across five stages; namely: (1) Denial: This happens in the very early phase of the dying process and represents the inability (or unwillingness) of the person to acknowledge that he or she is dying. This initial resistance to the reality that one is in the terminal stages of living is an important precursor to bringing one's own death into proper focus. Once a person acknowledges that he or she is, indeed, dying, the remaining stages can then present themselves into conscious awareness. (2) Anger: As life grows shorter, feelings of anger may emerge from the dying person. This form of penultimate anger could be directed at family, friends, professionals, or even oneself. A person may also experience nondiscriminant anger as he or she begins to realize that nothing can be done to stop the dying process. (3) Bargaining: This phase of the dying process describes a person's attempt to buy time. Bargaining is a manifestation of a latent hope for recovery or even the postponement of death. (4) Depression: Symptoms of depression are indicative of coming to grips with the reality of one's own dying. In this sense the experience of depression may include sadness, hopelessness, and other negative affective symptoms. However, such emotions are not necessarily pathological but predictable consequences of the person's ultimate fear of his or her own approaching death. (5) Acceptance: As death nears, the process of acceptance of this reality and of life review as a way of putting one's affairs in order (or to give life retrospective meaning) and letting go of old hurts and wounds occurs. This can have profound value, especially if the person is lucid enough to engage in these kinds of conscious recollections. Kübler-Ross's stages of dying culminate in a dignified death that occurs when the fully mature person accepts his or her ultimate end.

Kübler-Ross's stage theory of dying has strong intuitive appeal and these stages have been incorporated in a variety of approaches to grief counseling (Worden, 1991). There are, however, a number of limitations to construing the dying process as a series of stages based on content observation of a limited number of individuals as Kübler-Ross has done. First, the nature of the stages is dependent on self-reports from those patients who are able to describe their experiences. These are most likely patients who are younger, more verbally articulate, and more capable of describing their own internal emotional experience. It could be that such a stage model may be relevant only to a subset of dying persons who possess these kinds of personal characteristics and the intellectual capacity to articulate such issues while in the dying process.

For the older person, there are a number of challenges that may occur in later life that could make this kind of stage model approach to dying difficult to apply in counseling. First, age-related physiological deterioration is often confounded with diminished cognitive function. As this occurs, it can become harder to discern the internal and/or emotional forces that may be operating on a person as he or she nears the end of life. This has implications for counseling because cognitive impairment can make interventions that require capabilities such as memory (to engage reminiscence), abstract thinking (to be able to contemplate the end of one's own existence) or verbal ability (to facilitate interpersonal interchange with family and friends) less effective (Rentz, Krikorian, & Keys, 2004). Second, very old adults may find themselves dying in contexts outside of their home where family and friends are unavailable, particularly if the dying process is a protracted phenomenon that occurs in an extended care community. Further, because old age represents the phase of life during which a person is expected to die, the emotional intensity and effort to be with an older person (versus someone who is younger) during the process of dying may be intermittent, particularly if the facility in which the person is dying is geographically removed from family and friends. Despite these issues, the stage theory of dying provides a conceptual framework for understanding the needs of the older dying person.

A more contemporary approach to the stage model of dying has been proposed by Buckman (1993). Buckman's stages of dying are reduced to three; namely, an initial phase where the person acknowledges that he or she is dying, a chronic phase where the person deals with the predictable consequences of dying, including declines in physical, cognitive, and emotional functioning, and a final stage that involves accepting one's own death. This model suggests that the occurrence of the final stage (acceptance) may only be realized if the physical and intellectual state of the person allows him or her to grasp the experience of dying near its very end. For a person with dementia, only the first two stages are descriptive of the dying process. The utility of this model for the geriatric practitioner who is working with elderly dying patients is its focus on the person's emotional response to dying and how emotions change as a person nears his or her own death as opposed to how dying occurs and is interpreted by the person intellectually (Copp, 1998). This is a critical distinction for counseling given that helping the client manage his or her emotions throughout the process is paramount. Where confusion, delirium, or even dementia are present the nature of the person's self-reports may not be indicative of the person's actual dying experience.

A second conceptual approach to the dying process links it to specific psychological states or attitudes. This viewpoint of dying has been described in a number of ways; however, one common conceptualization is called "death anxiety" (Langs, 2004; Niemeyer, 1994) and underscores the anticipatory/affective component of death and dying that manifests itself in an emotional state (e.g., fear, anxiety, terror, dread, threat). The importance of emotional regulation is highlighted in this model of dying particularly as one nears the point of total loss of control. Some research has reported that aging, by itself, may be either unrelated or even inversely related to the trajectory of death anxiety; that is, among older adults who are relatively healthy, death anxiety may decrease with increasing age (Bengston, Cuellar, & Ragan, 1977).

In a contemporary meta-analytic review of factors that could influence the nature of death anxiety in old age, Fortner and Niemeyer (1999) reported that higher (or more pronounced) death anxiety was apparent among those persons who reported more health problems, were prone to distress, perceived themselves as more vulnerable and less resilient, and were more equivocal about their religious beliefs. These data underscore the complex nature of death anxiety in later life and the difficulty of pinpointing areas of fear and concern during the dying process. The death anxiety paradigm suggests that a dying person employs social and psychological mechanisms to deal with anticipatory anxiety and that if these coping mechanisms could be identified through an appropriate assessment mechanism, interventions tailored to the person's concerns could be developed.

The death anxiety model has a number of strengths for guiding counseling. First, unlike stage models, a relatively large literature has examined it across persons who vary with respect to individual characteristics, including age, gender, and ethnicity (Cicirelli, 1999; Niemeyer, Wittokowski, & Moser, 2004). In this sense, it is a model that can be applied to a wide range of older persons. Second, research has also documented that there are numerous strategies that people use to defend themselves against death anxiety, and these strategies, if identified, can be strengthened through counseling. One's religious or spiritual beliefs are a personal characteristic that could be a part of an intervention approach for dealing with the dying process and for alleviating anxiety. This is supported by surveys of older people near life's end who desire that health-care professionals attending to their needs address spiritual or religious issues (Ehman, Ott, Short, Ciampa, & Hansen-Flaschen, 1999). Given this scenario, it would be important for health-care providers who deal with end-of-life issues to be sensitive to spiritual or religious concerns of their dying patients and work collaboratively with clergy or spiritual leaders rather than simply refer these patients to members of the clergy or to those who are part of the patient's religious community. Third, the death anxiety conceptualization lends itself to interventions designed to diminish anxiety, fear, or the anticipation of threat. Stress inoculation therapy has been proposed in the clinical literature and could be useful in helping an older dying person find dignity in dying (Meichenbaum, 1996). In essence, stress inoculation therapy involves understanding the nature of the threat (in this case one's own death) and engaging in behaviors that prepare a person to meet that threat when it occurs (putting one's affairs in order, rallying social support, getting in touch with one's sense of meaning). Other therapy approaches that are more existential in nature and that work to alleviate anxiety can also be developed from this theoretical model (LeShan, 1969).

The weakness of the death anxiety model is its tendency to pathologize the dying process (e.g., that it is primarily associated with anxious/fearful affect). Similar to stage theories of dying, the basis for judging whether an older person is experiencing death anxiety is the presumption that cognitive functioning is intact. For older adults who have cognitive impairment it may not be possible to gauge their fear or anxiety about dying. Finally, it may be difficult in persons who have had a history of chronic anxiety or depression, to disentangle the cause of anxiety during the dying process. The question in the case of a person with a life history of depression or anxiety arises as to whether death anxiety is qualitatively different from clinical depression or pathological anxiety (Block, 2000).

These models of dying characterize the complexity of the interaction of psychological and physical forces as these influence an individual's response to the dying process, including the person's internal state (e.g., death anxiety) at qualitatively distinct points along a dying continuum (e.g., stages). These theoretically distinct approaches suggest, however, that coping with death involves engaging psychological mechanisms to deal, in a positive, dignified way, with anticipated changes in one's physical and psychological well-being that are precursors to the end of one's life.

Managing Emotions in Death and Dying

Both the stage and anxiety models of death and dying point to the management of emotions or the attributions associated with this process. The degree to which a person can regulate emotions through the dying process should predict whether he or she can continue to meaningfully relate to the world and to others up to life's end. With respect to positive aging, the recruitment of positive emotions may be helpful for some people to address the distress and discomfort that is likely in the dying experience; that is, the cultivation of a realistic, but optimistic appraisal of one's situation and needs, even if suffering near the end of life restricts the quality of day to day living.

Some research suggests that there may be multiple sources for positive emotions in the presence of dying (Field & Cassel, 1997). In fact, studies that have examined the role of positive emotions in mediating stress (Folkman, 1997) could have application to coping with the death and dying process. Several sources of positive emotions include: (1) *Family and loved ones:* For older adults, family may represent a meaningful extension of the life span, particularly younger members of one's social network, including children, grandchildren, nieces, and nephews. Not only can family relationships be a source of important interpersonal interchange during the dying process, their expressed memories and experiences of the older relative can be a source of shared pleasure. Further, younger members of the family are likely to carry with them the memory of the older dying relative, and in this sense, they may represent a source of legacy for the older person. (2) *Spiritual and religious beliefs:* Religious belief systems and spirituality represent an important source of meaning for many persons, and this has been documented by a plethora of research demonstrating the powerful buffering effects of spirituality and religious beliefs in times of stress (Cartwright, 1991; Sulmasy, 2002).There may also be, for the subset of persons who belong to organized religions, the comfort of rituals, rites, and social contact with clergy or religious leaders during the dying period. (3) *Social and personal values for living:* These values, although primarily connected to one's life-span belief system, can also be part of a person's sense of meaning irrespective of whether they espouse a religious belief system. Specifically, these are values that have facilitated the living of life in such a way as to bring them meaning. Several of these values were highlighted in Chapter 7 and include gratitude for one's life and the experiences that one has had across the course of life, and the relationships that have been a source of meaning. Forgiveness is another value that could be a potent source of positive emotions, particularly if there are opportunities to engage forgiveness at the end of life in order to get closure on unfinished *business*. For example, in a Gallup Poll (1997) that involved a telephone interview of a sample of 1200 adults, responding to questions indicating their greatest concern if they were dying, 72% reported that it would be knowing they had been forgiven by God, and just over 50% hoped that they would be reconciled with others. This underscores the prominence of forgiveness in dying a "good death" (Braun & Zir, 2001). Like forgiveness and gratitude, personal values for living can be a powerful source for maintaining a sense of continuity as one nears the end of life. The vignette below provides an example of how an older person might engage some of these sources of positive aging to optimize the dying process.

Gertrude was 94 years old and for most of her life lived in midtown Chicago. She was married for 50 years and had been a widow for 20 years, but had no children from the union. After the death of her husband, Gertrude made several investments in property that had substantially increased in value with the passage of time. Although Gertrude had a sizable net worth, most of her money was tied up in her property and investments. In her older years she became more reclusive and was nearly forgotten by extended family. When her health took a turn for the worse, she was taken to the hospital by a neighbor. At that time her old and frail condition precluded any medial intervention. Her attorney suggested a hospice because it was Gertrude's wish to spend her final years in her own home. The hospital had a well-developed hospice program, so Gertrude was released into her attorney's care and a nurse-practitioner who provided for hospice services was assigned to help Gertrude manage the dying process in Gertrude's own home. In visiting with the nurse-practitioner, Gertrude expressed an intense feeling of loneliness and feared dying alone and entirely forgotten by her family. Through the process of counseling, the nurse-practitioner felt that it might be helpful if Gertrude sent letters to relatives and friends who had received money from her in the past. She consented to engage this process and she dictated letters to the nurse-practitioner who then sent them to Gertrude's family members. It was not long before she received a number of phone calls, cards, and personal visits from family and friends. One family member took it upon herself to personally help Gertrude with putting her things in order before she died. Gertrude was pleased and accepted this family member's offer to help. In the intervening months, however, Gertrude's memory began slipping and she had difficulty interacting with the professional caregivers who were providing her with 24-hour care. She did, however, remember her sister, who was still living and who began visiting Gertrude when the sister received Gertrude's letter. Gertrude desired to be near her family at the time of her death, so several members of her family agreed to stay with her in her final hours. In the third month of hospice, her condition became worse and her pain medication was increased. Her breathing became labored and she slipped into a coma and died not long thereafter.

Gertrude's story highlights positive aging as a manifestation of a person's strategic use of his or her resources to optimize living. At the end of life, these resources are evaluated and readied to do the final work of living, which is to negotiate one's own exit from the world. Like other developmental tasks, this takes energy and effort. Therefore, an important aspect of positive aging is to be able to discuss the dying process openly with the dying person as well as her or his support network. If this occurs, it can lead to additional understanding about the needs of the dying person.

Steinhouser and colleagues interviewed terminally ill patients about their view of what they believed represented conditions that promoted the highest quality in relation to the dying process, or, positive aging in dying. From this research, five topics emerged (Steinhauser et al., 2000). They are (1) *Symptom and pain management:* The dying person wants not just to be pain free, but to manage pain in such a way that emotional and intellectual resources remain intact during the process of dying. (2) *Clarity of decision making:* The dying person wants to be involved in the decisions that are made about his or her care. In addition, the dying person's expressed need is to consider the concerns of his or her family and loved ones as well. (3) *Preparation for death:* The dying person needs time to make preparations for death. This may involve allowing the dying person to suffer and struggle with the process of dying versus being overmedicated as a way to avoid pain. (4) *Contribution to others:* It is important for the dying person to feel that he or she has contributed to the welfare of others. A positive aging approach to dying will address this important need. (5) *Affirmation of the whole person:* Even in death, the dying person requests that her or his rights and dignity are respected.

Embedded in these five principles is an approach to counseling that helps the person stay focused in the present in order to find peace in the process of dying. A support context built on these principles will help a person crystallize her or his own personal meaning and preserve positive aging even in dying.

The Role of the Professional Counselor

The professional counselor can play an important role in helping an older person negotiate the dying process in a number of ways. However, this role, for the most part, encompasses three areas of service provision: (1) assessment and identification of areas that could benefit from counseling; (2) helping the client manage the psychological or emotional experience of dying; (3) interfacing with the dying person's context including family, friends, and professional caregivers.

An important precursor to counseling persons who are dying is assessment. The purpose of assessment is twofold: (1) gauging the extent of distress the person is experiencing during the dying process and (2) identifying intrinsic resources that a person might recruit to facilitate coping (Niemeyer, 2001). High levels of anxiety or fear can limit a person's coping capacity during the dying process and make it difficult for caregivers to provide support and comfort. For this reason, the effective counselor should be aware, not only of the level of physical pain a dying person is experiencing at any given point in time, but also the degree to which a person is fearful, depressed, or anxious about dying (Block, 2000).

The easiest method for assessing anxiety or fear is to simply ask the dying person whether he or she is feeling anxious or afraid.

However, such a question may prove difficult to answer especially if the person is experiencing a range of conflicting emotions. Further, for the dying person who is attempting to control his or her emotional response, such an open-ended question might provoke an unnecessary negative emotional reaction. A more specific set of questions could provide a clearer direction for counseling interventions while at the same time minimizing the likelihood of catasrophizing on the part of the client. For example, if a dying older person is anxious about the unknown and fears losing control of his/her life, it may be useful to help the patient identify sources of personal belief or existential faith and explore how these might help to ameliorate fears (e.g., life after death). If however, a person is anxious about unfinished life business, the perspective of family or friends might help to alleviate such fears.

The scientific literature indicates that there are several areas where anxious affect is most likely to be experienced (Haley, Larson, Kasl-Godley, & Niemeyer, 2003). These are: (1) fear of pain and suffering associated with the dying process; (2) fear of loss of control; (3) unfinished business in life; (4) fear of the unknown (Niemeyer, 1994). An informal assessment might involve asking the dying patient if he or she is feeling troubled or anxious in these specific areas and, if so, what strategies that person is using to deal with those fears. To gauge severity, it might be useful to ask the person to rate the level of concern he or she has for each of these issues (mild, moderate, or severe). Such information could provide a starting point to develop an intervention that could address both the content of the anxiety, as well as the degree to which the person feels anxious about specific content.

For older adults the question of cognitive impairment might influence the nature of counseling. If one is dying and also cognitively impaired, counseling might emphasize the provision of physical comfort (soothing touch, music), as well as managing the concerns and fears of extended caregivers. For cognitively impaired older people, a focus on the here-and-now may be more beneficial than retrospective memories which could be distorted as a consequence of diminished long-term memory capacity (Trabert, 1996). Interestingly, some qualitative research has suggested that for cognitively impaired adults, the encouragement of emotional expression may be more problematic than helpful (Rentz et al., 2004). In contrast, for the cognitively impaired, the focus on acceptance of one's terminal condition (or even distraction away from thoughts of death) might be more therapeutic. To assess for cognitive problems, a simple mental status examination may be useful to employ. Several paper-and-pencil measures, such as the Pfeiffer Portable Mental Status Questionnaire, were presented in Chapter 4. In addition to mental status, the counselor should be aware of medications or palliative therapies that are currently being provided to the dying older person as these could also impact cognitive function and emotional regulation.

The second area of effective counseling is helping the client manage his or her emotions during the process of dying. This may involve not only the regulation of negative emotional states such as depression, anxiety, and fear, but also cultivating positive emotions as well. These strategies encourage the dying patient to reframe anxious or negative thoughts to those that focus on positive relational emotions (e.g., "I will never see my daughter again" to "The time I have left with my daughter is of great value to me"). Engaging the dying patient in the exploration of sources of happiness and well-being either in the past or the immediate present can have positive therapeutic benefits (Breitbart, Gibson, Poppito, & Berg, 2004). Two strategies from grief counseling literature have been suggested: (1) the use of life review to focus the patient on the positive memories in his or her past (Haight, 1988; Lichter, Mooney, & Boyd, 1993; Webster, 1995), and (2) The reframing of negative emotions using here-and-now strategies (Chocinov, 2002). This latter approach encourages the dying client to focus selectively on the moment. For example, the counselor can engage the dying person in a dialogue that focuses on the beauty of the flowers that are sitting on the table, the specific meaning of a story or a poem that is being read in his or her immediate presence, or the pleasurable aspects of his or her care (e.g., bathing, a massage). The goal of the here-and-now is to optimize self-control. This strategy may also have value for the cognitively impaired older person who may have difficulty contemplating the past or the future due to impaired intellectual functioning.

A third area of effective counseling is meaningfully interfacing with the context in which the dying person resides. These are often settings removed from the home environment. The National Hospice and Palliative Care Organization (2001) has estimated that approximately 25% of the elderly in the United States die at home in contrast to 50% who die in hospital settings and 25% who die in nursing home or long-term care facilities. These data indicate that in contemporary society, for most people who live into very old age the likelihood is high that they will die away from their own home environment. Interestingly, research suggests that older persons, if given a preference, would prefer to die at home (Ben-Klug, Gessert, & Forbes, 2001). For these reasons, the experience of dying in a hospital facility or nursing home may exacerbate one's anticipatory fear of death and make it difficult to cultivate positive emotions in unfamiliar contexts. This phenomenon has prompted institutional facilities and advocates for the dying to develop models of end-of-life care that are more conducive to a context that maximizes quality of life and well-being during the dying process.

Hospice Care as an Example of Positive Aging in Dying

The notion of hospice comes from the centuries old idea of offering a place of shelter or "hospitality" to weary or sick travelers. A contemporary definition of hospice that underscores this notion from *Webster's New World Dictionary* is: "A home-like facility for care of a terminally ill patient." In addition to a "place" to die, hospice also represents a way of thinking about dying that affirms the rights to quality of life for a dying person through a humane form of care that is focused on the qualitative aspects of dying as opposed to strategies or techniques to maintain life at any cost. Therefore, the idea of hospice encompasses both a context and a philosophy of dying.

A term that is useful in elucidating the characteristics of hospice care is the idea of *dying in place* or dying in a way that is consistent with the expressed wishes of the patient. In this sense, hospice tries to create a homelike environment for the patient even though the person who is dying may be in an institutional setting. If it is in a hospital setting, for example, once hospice has been enacted, decisions about life-sustaining equipment and technology are reevaluated from the viewpoint of preserving the quality of life and the dignity of the individual in his or her final stage of life.

There are a number of objectives that hospice works toward and a "best practices" approach to hospice care should provide: (1) A professional to manage the dying patient's general health needs. Because hospice is a combination of many different services, a case manager usually develops a hospice care plan. (2) Strategies for symptom and pain relief. This includes close monitoring of the patient's vital signs and the use of medication and psychological strategies to diminish pain and discomfort. (3) The provision of ongoing personal care assistance. This could include help for activities such as bathing, toileting, and dressing. This might also involve more complex tasks such as helping the patient put his or her affairs in order by making contact with family and friends through phone calls or letters. (4) A way to address the emotional and existential needs of the dying patient. Hospice workers should be trained to listen, support, and care while at the same time respecting the personal beliefs of the client. (5) Ongoing bereavement and grief counseling to the patient and the patient's immediate family or close loved ones. An important role and function of hospice counselors is to help prepare the family to deal with their grief before and after the death of the patient.

Hospice (National Hospice & Palliative Care Organization, 2000) integrates a number of dimensions of care that are consistent with positive aging including: affirming the positive nature of life even at its end; not attempting to hasten or postpone death, rather, meeting the diversity of needs expressed by the dying patient; treating the person rather than the disease including emphasizing both the physical and emotional needs of the dying person; a focus on quality of life, not curing illness, as the goal, providing comfort and positive reassurance by way of a family-centered approach to care that involves an ongoing dialogue with the dying patient, the family, and the health-care provider (Chocinov, 2002).

Most older people who are in the final stages of life want to optimize their level of comfort through palliative care that emphasizes medications and treatment to control pain and maximize comfort (Emanual & Emanual, 1998). At the same time, the older person who is struggling to maintain cognitive coherence due to heavy pain medication regimens may also want to preserve his or her awareness and conscious functioning for as long as possible. Among older dying patients who are at risk for cognitive decline, medication management must balance these contrasting needs (Haley et al., 2003).

In an illuminating qualitative study that examined the experience of dying in a nursing home context Kayser-Jones (2002) highlighted the importance of humanizing the dying process even for persons who are not cognitively aware, as is the case in persons suffering from dementia. In her description of how staff interacted with nursing home residents who were at various stages of dying, those behaviors that affirmed the individual by respecting his or her remaining capabilities were associated with positive emotional outcomes. Those patient–staff interactions that tended to ignore individual differences (including intact skills and functionality), and that were designed to maximize systemic efficiency at the expense of individual needs, were uniformly viewed by the patient and the patient's loved ones as insensitive and, in some cases, deleterious. Her research suggests that care institutions for the elderly should avoid making implicit assumptions about residents ("This person is memory impaired so he doesn't need to be asked if he is ready for dinner."), but should engage careful assessment to determine the objective strengths and weaknesses of the individual. Therefore, for hospice to promote positive aging it must provide a form of care that is consistent with the unique psychosocial, cultural, and spiritual needs of the dying patient regardless of the context in which they are dying.

CONCLUDING COMMENTS

This chapter has examined the nature of loss from two perspectives; namely, the loss of loved ones through death and the experience of loss associated with one's own dying. In both instances positive aging can be a source of coping. Two areas were highlighted as coping resources: (1) one's social network and the encouragement it provides with respect to the loss, and (2) the reframing of loss through the cultivation of positive emotions. The role of the professional counselor as an active agent who engages these kinds of positive aging strategies to address the issues of loss was described. Key roles for the professional counselor can be found in assessment, intervention planning, and implementation of intervention approaches that promote positive aging. Effective counseling strategies capitalize on the strengths inherent within the individual and in his or her social network as these are engaged to cope with loss-related challenges. Hospice was presented as an example of a positive aging approach to the needs of dying person.

BIBLIOGRAPHY

AARP (2001). *Caregiver identification study.* Washington, DC: Author. American Association of Retired Persons.

Abeles, N., Victor, T. L., & Delano-Wood, L. (2004). The impact of an older adult's death on the family. *Psychology & Aging, 35*(3), 234–239.

Adler, A. (1937). Mass psychology. *International Journal of Individual Psychology, 2,* 64–68.

Aerán, P. A. (2003). Advances in psychotherapy for mental illness in late life. *American Journal of Geriatric Psychiatry, 11,* 4–6.

Albert, M. S., Jones, K., Savage, C. R., Berkman, L., Seeman, T., Blazer, D., Rowe, J. W. (1995). Predictors of cognitive change in older persons: MacArthur studies of successful aging. *Psychology & Aging, 10*(4), 578–589.

Alexopoulos, G. S., Abrams, R., Young, R., & Shamoian, C. (1988a). Cornell scale for depression in dementia. *Biological Psychiatry, 23*(3), 271–284.

Alexopoulos, G. S., Abrams, R. C., Young, R. C., & Shamoian, C. A. (1988b). Use of the Cornell scale in nondemented patients. *Journal of the American Geriatric Society, 36,* 230–236.

Alpert, M. J. (1994). *The chronically disabled elderly in society.* Westport, CT: Greenwood Press.

Altschuler, J., Katz, A. D., & Tynan, M. (2004). Developing and implementing an HIV/AIDS educational curriculum for older adults. *Gerontologist, 44*(1), 121–126.

American Psychological Association (2004). Guidelines for psychological practice with older adults. *American Psychologist, 59*(4), 236–260.

Bibliography

Alzheimer's Association (1995). Giving up the car keys. *National Newsletter, 3*(1), 7.

American Psychiatric Association. (1994). *Diagnostic and statistical manual of mental disorders* (4th ed.). Washington, DC: Author.

Andres, R. (1985). Normal aging versus disease in the elderly. In R. Andres, E. L. Bierman, & W. R. Hazzard (Eds.), *Principles of geriatric medicine* (pp. 38–41). New York: McGraw-Hill.

Anthony, J. C., & Aboraya, A. (1992). The epidemiology of selected mental disorders in later life. In J. E. Birren, R. B. Sloane, G. D. Cohen, N. R. Hooyman, B. Leibowitz, & M. H. Wykle (Eds.), *Handbook of mental health and aging* (2nd ed., pp. 27–73). San Diego, CA: Academic Press.

Anthony, J. C., LeResche, L., Niaz, U., von Korff, M. R., & Folstein, M. F. (1982). Limits of the "Mini-Mental State" as a screening test for dementia and delirium among hospital patients. *Psychological Medicine, 12,* 397–408.

Antonucci, T. C. (2000). Statements from the candidates for presidency of GSA. *Gerontology News,* April 5, 5.

Aranda, M. P., Villa, V. M., Trejo, L. R., Ramirez, R., & Ranney, M. (2003). El Portal Latino Alzheimer's Project: Model program for Latino caregivers of Alzheimer's disease-affected people. *Social Work, 48,* 259–271.

Arbuckle, T. Y., Gold, D. P., Andres, D., Schwartzman, A. E., & Chaikelson, J. (1992). The role of psychosocial context, age, and intelligence in memory performance of older men. *Psychology & Aging, 7,* 25–36.

Ardelt, M. (1997). Wisdom and life satisfaction in old age. *Journals of Gerontology: Psychological and Social Sciences, 52*(1), 15–27.

Aréan, P. A. (2003). Advances in psychotherapy for mental illness in late life. *American Journal of Geriatric Psychiatry, 11,* 4–6.

Arking, R. (1998). *Biology of aging: Observations and principles.* Sunderland, MA: Sinauer Associates.

Atchley, R. C. (1989). A continuity theory of normal aging. *Gerontologist, 29*(2), 183–190.

Bäckman, L., & Dixon, R. (1992). Psychological compensation: A theoretical framework. *Psychological Bulletin, 112,* 259–283.

Bäckman, L., Josephsson, S., Herlitz, A., Stigsdotter, A., & Uiitanen, M. (1991). The generalizability of training gains in dementia: Effects of an imagery based mnemonic on face-name retention duration. *Psychology & Aging, 6,* 489–492.

Bailey, D., & McNally, K. K. (1996). Interorganizational community-based collaboratives: A strategic response to shape the social work agenda. *Social Work, 41,* 602–611.

Baker, J. L. (1958). The unsuccessful aged. *Journal of the American Geriatrics Society, 7,* 570–572.

Baltes, M. M. (1995). Dependency in old age: Gains and losses. *Current Directions in Psychological Science, 4,* 14–19.

Baltes, P. B. (1993). The aging mind: Potential and limits. *Gerontologist, 33*(5), 580–594.

Baltes, P. B. (1997). On the incomplete architecture of human ontogeny: Selection, optimization, and compensation as foundation of developmental theory. *American Psychologist, 52,* 366–380.

Baltes, P. B., & Baltes, M. M. (1990). Psychological perspectives on successful aging: The model of selective optimization with compensation. In P. B. Baltes & M. M. Baltes (Eds.), *Successful aging: Perspectives from the behavioral sciences* (pp. 1–34). Cambridge, MA: Cambridge University Press.

Baltes, P. B., Baltes, M. M., Freund, A. M., & Lang, F. R. (1995). *Measurement of selective optimization with compensation by questionnaire.* Berlin, Germany: Max Planck Institute for Human Development.

Baltes, P. B., Baltes, M. M., Freund, A. M., & Lang, F. R. (1999). *The measurement of selection, optimization, and compensation (SOC) by self report.* Berlin, Germany: Max Planck Institute for Human Development.

Baltes, P. B., Dittmann-Kohli, F., & Kliegl, R. K. (1986). Reserve capacity of the elderly in aging-sensitive tests of fluid intelligence: Replication and extension. *Psychology & Aging, 1,* 172–177.

Baltes, P. B., & Staudinger, U. M. (2000). Wisdom: A metaheuristic (pragmatic) to orchestrate mind and virtue toward excellence. *American Psychologist, 55*(1), 122–135.

Baltes, P. B., Staudinger, U. M., & Lindenberger, U. (1999). Lifespan psychology: Theory and application to intellectual functioning. *Annual Review of Psychology, 51,* 471–507.

Baltes, P. B., Staudinger, U. M., Maercker, A., & Smith, J. (1995a). People nominated as wise: A comparative study of wisdom-related knowledge. *Psychology & Aging, 10*(2), 155–166.

Baltes, P. P., Staudinger, U. M., Maercker, A., & Smith, J. (1995b). The search for the psychology of wisdom. *Current Directions in Psychological Science, 2,* 75–80.

Bankoff, E. (1983). Social support and adaptation to widowhood. *Journal of Marriage and the Family, 45,* 827–839.

Barnes, C. A. (1998). Memory changes during normal aging: Neurobiological correlates. In J. L. Martinez & R. P. Kesner (Eds.), *Neurobiology of Learning and Memory* (pp. 247–287). New York: Academic Press.

Barusch, A. S., Rogers, A., & Abu-Bader, S. (1999). Depressive symptoms among the frail elderly: Physical and psycho-social correlates. *International Journal of Aging and Human Development, 49*(2), 107–125.

Barusch, A. S., & Spaid, W. M. (1996). Spouse caregivers and the caregiving experience: Does cognitive impairment make a difference? *Journal of Gerontological Social Work, 25,* 93–105.

Beach, S. R., Schulz, R., Yee, J. L., & Jackson, S. (2000). Negative and positive health effects of caring for a disabled spouse: Longitudinal findings from the caregiver health effects study. *Psychology & Aging, 15* (2), 259–271.

Bédard, M., Molloy, D. W., Squire, L., Dubois, S., Lever, J. A., & O'Donnell, M. (2001). The Zarit Burden Interview: A new short version and screening version. *Gerontologist, 41*(5), 652–657.

Beekman, A. T. F., Deeg, D. J. H., Van Tilberg, T., Smit, J. H., Hooijer, C., & Van Tilberg, W. (1995). Major and minor depression in later life: A study of prevalence and risk factors. *Journal of Affective Disorders, 36,* 65–75.

Bem, D. J. (1970). *Beliefs, attitudes and human affairs.* Belmont, CA: Brooks-Cole.

Benbow, S. M. & Marriott, A. (1997). Family therapy with elderly people. *Advances in Psychiatric Treatment, 3,* 138–145.

Bengston, V. L., Cuellar, J. B., & Ragan, P. K. (1977). Stratum contrasts and similarities in attitudes toward death. *Journal of Gerontology, 32,* 76–88.

Ben-Klug, M., Gessert, C., & Forbes, S. (2001). The need to revise assuptions about the end of life: Implications for social work practice. *Health and Social Work, 26* (1), 38–48.

Berkman, L., Berkman, C., & Kasl, S. (1986). Depressive symptoms in relation to physical health and functioning in the elderly. *American Journal of Epidemiology, 124,* 372–388.

Berkman, L. F., Seeman, T. E., Albert, M. S., Blazer, D., Kahn, R., Mohs, R., Finch, C., et al. (1993). Successful, usual and impaired functioning in community dwelling elderly: MacArthur Successful Aging Field Studies. *Journal of Clinical Epidemiology, 46,* 1129–1140.

Bickenbach, J. E., Chatterji, S., Badley, E. M., & Ustun, T. B. (1999). Models of disablement, universalism and the international classification of impairments, disabilities and handicaps. *Social Science Medicine, 48,* 1173–1187.

Black, H. K., & Rubinstein, R. L. (2004). Themes of suffering in later life. *Journal of Gerontology: Psychological and Social Sciences, 59,* 17–24.

Blazer, D. G. (2003). Depression in late life: Review and commentary. *Journal of Gerontology: Biological and Medical Sciences, 58,* 249–265.

Blazer, D. G., Hays, J. C., Fillenbaum, G. G., & Gold, D. T. (1997). Memory complaint as a predictor of cognitive decline: A comparison of African American and white elders. *Journal of Aging and Health, 9,* 171–184.

Block, S. D. (2000). Assessing and managing depression in the terminally ill patient. *Annals of Internal Medicine, 132,* 209–218.

Boerner, K. (2004). Adaptation to disability among middle-aged and older adults: The role of assimilative and accommodative coping. *Journal of Gerontology: Psychological Sciences, 59* (1), 34–42.

Boland, A., & Cappeliez, P. (1997). Optimism and neuroticism as predictors of coping and adaptation in older women. *Personality and Individual Differences, 22* (6), 909–919.

Bolla, K., Lindgren, K. N., Bonaccorsy, C., & Bleecker, L. (1991). Memory complaints in older adults: Fact or fiction? *Archives of Neurology, 48,* 61–64.

Boller, F., & Katzman, R. (1989). *Biological markers of Alzheimer's disease.* New York: Springer Verlag.

Bonanno, G. A. (1999). Laughter during bereavement. *Bereavement Care, 18,* 19–22.

Bonanno, G. A., & Kaltman, S. (1999). Toward an integrative perspective on bereavement. *Psychological Bulletin, 125,* 760–776.

Bonanno, G. A., Papa, A., O'Neil, K., Westphal, M. & Coifman, K. (2004). The importance of being flexible: The ability to enhance and supress emotional expression predicts long-term adjustment. *Psychological Science, 15,* 482–487.

Bonanno, G. A., Wortman, C. B., & Nesse, R. M. (2004). Prospective patterns of resilience and maladjusment during widowhood. *Psychology & Aging, 19* (2), 260–271.

Bond, J. (1982). Volunteering and life satisfaction among older adults. *Canadian Counsellor, 16,* 168–172.

Borkovec, T. D., Schadick, R. N., & Hopkins, M. (1991). The nature of normal and pathological worry. In R. M. Rapee & D. H. Barlow (Eds.), *Chronic anxiety: Generalized anxiety disorder and mixed anxiety-depression.* New York: Guilford Press.

Botwinick, J. (1966). Cautiousness in advanced age. *Journal of Gerontology, 21,* 347–353.

Botwinick, J. (1969). Disinclination to venture response versus cautiousness in responding: Age differences. *Journal of Genetic Psychology, 115,* 55–62.

Bradford, J., Caitlin, R., & Rothblum, E. D. (1994). National lesbian health care survey 7: Implications for mental health care. *Journal of Consulting and Clinical Psychology, 62*(2), 228–242.

Bradley, E. H., Fried, T. R., Kasl, S. V., & Idler, E. (2000). Quality-of-life trajectories of elders in the end of life. *Annual Review of Gerontology and Geriatrics, 20,* 64–96.

Braithwaite, V. (2002). Reducing ageism. In T. D. Nelson (Ed.), *Ageism, stereotyping, & prejudice against older persons.* Cambridge, MA: MIT Press. (pp. 311–388).

Brandsma, J. M. (1982). Forgiveness: A dynamic, theological and theoretical analysis. *Pastoral Psychology, 31,* 40–50.

Brandtstedter, J. (1990). Tenacious goal pursuit and flexible goal adjustment: Explication and age-related analysis of assimilative and accommodative strategies of coping. *Psychology & Aging, 5,* 58–67.

Braun, K. L., & Zir, A. (2001). Roles for the church in improving end-of-life care: Perceptions of Christian clergy and laity. *Death Studies, 25* (8), 685–704.

Bravo, G., Gauthier, P., Roy, P. M., Payette, H., Gaulin, P., Harvey, M., & Peloquin, L. (1996). Impact of a 12-month exercise program on the physical and psychological health of osteopenic women. *Journal of the American Geriatrics Society, 44* (7), 756–762.

Breitbart, W., Gibson, C., Poppito, S. R., & Berg, A. (2004). Psychotherapy interventions at the end of life: A focus on meaning and spirituality. *Canadian Journal of Psychiatry, 49,* 366–372.

Broerner, K., Schulz, R., & Horowitz, A. (2004). Positive aspects of caregiving and adaption to bereavement. *Psychology & Aging, 19*(4), 668–675.

Brown, L. B., & Ott, R. R. (2004). Driving and dementia: A review of the literature. *Journal of Geriatric Psychiatry and Neurology, 17*(4), 232–240.

Brangman, S. A., Espino, D. V., Goldstein, M. K., McCabe, M., Reed, R., Tylenda, C. (2003). *American Geriatrics Society (AGS) position statement on ethnogeriatrics.* AGS, New York: NY.

Buckman, R. (2001). Communication skills in palliative care: A practical guide. *Neurology & Clinical Neurology, 19,* 989–1004.

Burlingame, G. M., Fuhriman, A., & Mosier, J. (2003). The differential effectiveness of group psychotherapy a meta-analytic perspective. *Group Dynamics: Theory, Research, and Practice, 7*(1), 3–12.

Burlingame, G. M., MacKenzie, K. R., & Strauss, B. (2004). Small-group treatment: Evidence for effectiveness and mechanisms of change. In M. J. Lambert (Ed.), *Handbook of psychotherapy and behavior change* (pp. 647–696). New York: Wiley.

Butler, R. (1963). The life review: An interpretation of reminiscence in the aged. *Psychiatry, 26,* 65–76.

Butler, R. (1974). Successful aging and the role of life review. *Journal of the American Geriatric Society, 22,* 529–535.

Camp, C. J., & Stevens, A. B. (1990). Spaced retrieval: A memory intervention for dementia of the Alzheimer's type (DAT). *Clinical Gerontologist, 10,* 58–61.

Carstensen, L. L. (1992). Social and emotional patterns in adulthood: Support for socioemotional selectivity theory. *Psychology & Aging, 7* (3), 331–338.

Cartwright, A. (1991). Is religion a help around the time of death? *Public Health, 105,* 79–87.

Cheng, C. (2001). Assessing coping flexibility in real-life and laboratory settings: A multimethod approach. *Journal of Personality & Social Psychology, 80,* 814–833.

Chocinov, H. M. (2002). Dignity-conserving care—A new model for palliative care. *Journal of the American Medical Association, 287*(17), 2253–2260.

Chou, K. L., & Chi, I. (2001). Selection, optimization, and compensation questionnaire: A validation study with Chinese older adults. *Clinical Gerontologist, 24,* 141–151.

Christensen, H. (1991). The validity of memory complaints by elderly persons. *International Journal of Geriatric Psychiatry, 6,* 307–312.

Christensen, H., MacKinnon, A., Korten, A., Jorm, A. F., Henderson, A., Jacomb, S. et al. (1999). An analysis of diversity in the cognitive performance of elderly community dwellers: Individual differences in change scores as a function of age. *Psychology & Aging, 14,* 365–379.

Cicirelli, V. G. (1999). Personality and demographic factors in older adults' fear of death. *Gerontologist, 39,* 569–579.

Cignac, M. A. M., Cott, C., & Badley, E. M. (2002). Applying selective optimization with compensation to the behaviors of older adults with osteoarthritis. *Psychology & Aging, 17*(3), 520–524.

Clayton, P. J. (1979). The sequelae and nonsequelae of conjugal bereavement. *American Journal of Psychiatry, 136,* 1530–1534.

Clegg, A., Bryant, J., Nicholson, T., McIntyre, L. M., De Broe, S., Gerard, K., et al. (2001). Clinical and cost-effectiveness of donepezil, revastigmine and galantamine for Alzheimer's disease: A rapid and systematic review. *High Technology Assessment, 5*(1), 1–143.

CNN. (1997). *World's oldest person dies at 122,* CNN Interactive. From http://www.cnn.com/WORLD/9708/04/obit.oldest/

Cockrell, J. R., & Folstein, M. F. (1988). Mini Mental State Examination (MMSE). *Psychopharmacology Bulletin, 24,* 689–692.

Cohen, C. I. (1999). Aging and homelessness. *Gerontologist, 39*(1), 5–14.

Cohen, C. I., Ramirez, M., Teresi, J., Gallagher, M., & Sokolovsky, J. (1997). Predictors of becoming redomiciled among older homeless women. *Gerontologist, 37*(1), 67–74.

Coles, L. S. (2004a). Demographics of human supercentenarians and the implications for longevity medicine. *Annals of the New York Academy of Sciences Online, 1019* (June), 490–495.

Coles, L. S. (2004b). Demography of supercentenarians. *Journal of Gerontology: Biological Sciences, 59*(6), 579–586.

Cooley, S., Deitch, I. M., Harper, M. S., Hinrichsen, G., Lopez, M. A., & Molinari, V. A. (1998). What practitioners should know about working with older adults. *Professional Psychology: Research and Practice, 29* (5), 413–427.

Coon, D. W., Rider, K., Gallagher-Thompson, D., & Thompson, L. (1999). Cognitive-behavioral therapy for the treatment of late-life distress. In M. Duffy (Ed.), *Handbook of counseling and psychotherapy with older adults* (pp. 487–510). New York: John Wiley.

Copp, G. (1998). A review of current theories of death and dying. *Journal of Advanced Nursing, 28,* 382–390.

Costa, P. T., & McCrae, R. R. (1986). Personality stability and its implications for clinical psychology. *Clinical Psychology Review, 6,* 407–423.

Costa, P. T. J., & McCrae, R. R. (1988). Personality in adulthood: A six-year longitudinal study of self-reports and spouse ratings on the NEO Personality Inventory. *Journal of Personality & Social Psychology, 54*(5), 853–863.

Costa, P. T., & McCrae, R. R. (1992a). Normal personality assessment in clinical practice: The NEO Personality Inventory. *Psychological Assessment, 4,* 5–13.

Costa, P. T. J., & McCrae, R. R. (1992b). *Revised NEO Personality Inventory professional manual.* Odessa, FL: Psychological Assessment Resources.

Cowley, M. (1980). *The view from 80.* New York: Viking Press.

Craik, F. I. M., Anderson, N. D., Kerr, S. A., & Li, K. A. H. (1995). Memory changes in normal aging. In A. D. Baddeley, B. A. Wilson & F. N. Watts (Eds.), *Handbook of memory disorders* (pp. 211–241). New York: John Wiley.

Crane, M. (1999). *Understanding older homeless people: Their circumstances, problems, and needs.* Buckingham, UK: Open University Press.

Craske, M. G., Barlow, D. H., & O'Leary, T. A. (1992). *Mastery of your anxiety and worry.* Albany, NY: Graywind.

Crits-Chistoph, P., & Barber, J. P. (1991). *Handbook of short-term dynamic psychotherapy.* New York: Basic.

Crook, T., Bartus, R. T., Ferris, S. H., Whitehouse, P., Cohen, G. D., & Gershon, S. (1986). Age-associated memory impariment: Proposed diagnostic criteria and measures of clinical change: Report of a National Institute of Mental Health Work Group. *Developmental Neuropsychology, 14,* 327–339.

Crowther, M. R., Parker, M. W., Achenbaum, W. A., Larimore, W. L., & Koenig, H. G. (2002). Rowe and Kahn's model of successful aging revisited: Positive spirituality—the forgotten factor. *Gerontologist, 42*(5), 613–620.

Crumbaugh, J., & Maholick, L. (1964). *Purpose in life test.* Murfreesboro, TN: Psychometric Affiliates.

Csernansky, J. G., Miller, J. P., McKeel, D., & Morris, J. C. (2002). Relationships among cerebrospinal fluid biomarkers in dementia of the Alzheimer type. *Alzheimer Disease & Associated Disorders, 16*(3), 144–149.

Csikszentmihalyi, M. (1990). *Flow: The psychology of optimal human experience.* New York: Harper & Row.

Cutler, D. (2001). The reduction of disability among the elderly. *Proceedings of the National Academy of Sciences, 98*(12), 6546–6547.

Czaja, S. J., Schulz, R., Chin Lee, C., & Belle, S. H. (2003). A methodology for describing and decomposing complex psychosocial and behavioral interventions. *Psychology & Aging, 18,* 385–389.

Davidowitz, M., & Myrick, R. D. (1984). Responding to the bereaved: An analysis of "helping" statements. *Psychological Record, 1*, 35–42.

Daviglus, M. L., Liu, K., Pirzada, A., Yan, L. L., Garside, D. B., Feinglass, J. et al. (2003). Favorable cardiovascular risk profile in middle age and health-related quality of life in older age. *Archives of Internal Medicine, 163*(20), 2460–2468.

Davis, H., & Rockwood, K. (2004). Conceptualization of mild cognitive impairment: A review. *International Journal of Geriatric Psychiatry, 19*(4), 313–319.

Deegear, J., & Lawson, D. M. (2003). The utility of empirically supported treatments. *Professional Psychology: Research and Practice, 34*(3), 271–277.

Deneberg, R. (1997). HIV infection in women: Still untreated, still deadly. *Treatment Issues, 7*, 1–4.

Derogatis, L. R., & Melisaratos, N. (1983). The brief symptom inventory: An introductory report. *Psychological Medicine, 13*(3), 595–605.

Diener, E. (2000). Subjective well-being: The science of happiness and a proposal for a national index. *American Psychologist, 55*, 34–43.

Diener, E., & Diener, C. (1996). Most people are happy. *Psychological Science, 7*, 181–185.

Diener, E., Emmons, R. A., Larson, R. J., & Griffin, S. (1985). The satisfaction with life scale. *Journal of Personality Assessment, 49*, 71–75.

Dobson, K. S. (2000). *Handbood of cognitive-behavioral therapies* (2nd ed.). New York: Guilford Press.

Doolin, J. (1986). Planning for the special needs of the homeless elderly. *Gerontologist, 26*, 229–231.

Drewnowski, A. & Schultz, J. M. (2001). Impact of aging on eating behaviors, food choices, nutrition, a health status. *Journal of Nutrition Health and Aging, 5*, 75–79.

Duchek, J. M., Carr, D. B., Hunt, L., Roe, C. M., Xiong, C., Shah, K. et al. (2003). Longitudinal driving performance in early-stage dementia of the Alzheimer type. *Journal of the American Geriatrics Society, 51*, 1342–1347.

Duffy, M. (1999). *Handbook of counseling and psycholotherapy with older adults*. New York: John Wiley.

Dulin, P., Hill, R. D., Anderson, J., & Rasmussen, D. (2001). Altruism as a predictor of life satisfaction in a sample of low-income older adult service providers. *Journal of Mental Health and Aging, 7*(3), 349–359.

Ehman, J. W., Ott, B. B., Short, T. H., Ciampa, R. C., & Hansen-Flaschen, J. (1999). Do patients want physicians to inquire about their spiritual or religious beliefs if they become gravely ill? *Archives of Internal Medicine, 159*, 1803–1806.

Ellis, A. (1987). The impossibility of achieving consistently good mental health. *American Psychologist, 42*(4), 364–375.

Emanual, E. J., & Emanual, L. L. (1998). The promise of a good death. *The Lancet, 351,* 21–29.

Emmons, R. A., & McCullough, M. E. (2003). Counting blessings versus burdens: An experimental investigation of gratitude and subjective well-being in daily life. *Journal of Personality and Social Psychology, 84*(2), 377–389.

Emmons, R. A., & McCullough, M. E. (2004). *The psychology of gratitude.* Cambridge, New York: Oxford University Press.

Endicott, J., & Spitzer, R. L. (1978). A diagnostic interview: The schedule for affective disorders and schizophrenia. *Archives of General Psychiatry, 35*(7), 837–844.

Engle, L. (1998). Old AIDs. *The Body Positive, 9,* 14–21.

Enright, R. D. (1991). The moral development of forgiveness. In W. Kurtines & J. Gewirtz (Eds.), *Moral behavior and development* (Vol. 1, pp. 123–152). Hillsdale, NJ: Erlbaum.

Enright, R. D., & Coyle, C. T. (1994). Researching the process model of forgiveness with psychological interventions. In E. L. Worthington (Ed.), *Dimensions of forgiveness* (pp. 139–162). Philadelphia, PA: Templeton Foundation Press.

Enright, R. D., & Fitzgibbons, R. P. (2000). *Helping clients forgive.* Washington, DC: American Psychological Association.

Erikson, E. H. (1963). *Childhood and society.* New York: W. W. Norton.

Erikson, E. H. (1968). *Identity youth and crisis.* New York: W. W. Norton.

Erikson, E. H. (1980). *Identity and the life cycle.* New York: W. W. Norton.

Erikson, E. H., Erikson, J. M., & Kivnick, H. O. (1986). *Vital involvement in old age.* New York: W. W. Norton.

Farlow, M., Anand, R., Messina, J., Hartman, R., & Veach, J. (2000). A 52-week study of the efficacy of rivastigmine in patients with mild to moderately severe Alzheimer's disease. *European Neurology, 44,* 236–241.

Faschingbauer, T. R., Zisook, S., & DeVaul, R. (1987). The Texas revised inventory of grief. In S. Zisook (Ed.), *Biopsychosocial aspects of bereavement.* Washington, DC: American Psychiatric Press.

Federal Interagency Forum on Aging Related Statistics (2001). *Older Americans 2000: Key indicators of well-being.* Washington, DC: Author.

Fenwick, R., & Barresi, C. M. (1981). Health consequences of marital-status change among the elderly: A comparison of cross-sectional and longitudinal analyses. *Journal of Health and Social Behavior, 22,* 106–116.

Field, M. J., & Cassel, C. K. (1997). *Approaching death: Improving care at the end-of-life.* Washington, DC: National Academy Press.

Fleg, J. L., & Lakatta, E. G. (1986). Cardiovascular disease in old age. In I. Rossman (Ed.), *Clinical geriatrics* (pp. 169–196). Philadelphia, PA: J. B. Lippincott.

Fleming, S., & Robinson, P. (2001). Grief and cognitive-behavioral therapy: The reconstruction of meaning. In M. S. Stroebe & R. O. Hansson (Eds.), *Handbook of bereavement research: Consequences, coping, and care.* (pp. 647–669). Washington, DC: American Psychological Association.

Florsheim, M. J., & Herr, J. J. (1990). Family counseling with elders. *Generations, 14,* 40–42.

Folkman, S. (1997). Positive psychological states and coping with severe stress. *Social Science Medicine, 45,* 1207–1221.

Folstein, M. F., Folstein, S. E., & McHugh, P. R. (1975). "Mini-Mental State": A practical method for grading the cognitive state of patients for the clinician. *Journal of Psychiatry Research, 12,* 189–198.

Fortner, B. V. & Niemeyer, R. A. (1999). Death anxiety in older adults: A quantitative review. *Death Studies, 23,* 387–411.

Frankl, V. E. (1985). *Psychotherapy and existentialism: Selected papers on logotherapy.* New York: Pocket.

Fredrickson, L. (2000). Cultivating positive emotions to optimize health and well-being. *Prevention and Treatment, 3,* 1–25.

Freedman, S. R., & Enright, R. D. (1996). Forgiveness as an intervention goal with incest survivors. *Journal of Consulting and Clinical Psychology, 64*(5), 983–992.

Freud, S. (1953). *On psychotherapy.* In James Strachey (Trans. & Ed.), *The standard edition of the complete psychological works of Sigmund Freud* (Vol. 7, pp. 255–268). Toronto, Canada: Hogarth Press. (Original work published 1905.)

Freund, A., Alexandra, M., & Baltes, P. B. (1998). Selection, optimization, and compensation as strategies of life management: Correlations with subjective indicators of successful aging. *Psychology & Aging, 13*(4), 531–543.

Freund, A. M., & Baltes, P. B. (2002). Life-management strategies of selection, optimization, and compensation: Measurement by self-report and construct validity. *Journal of Personality and Social Psychology, 82*(4), 642–662.

Freund, A. M., Li, Z. H., & Baltes, P. B. (1999). The role of selection, optimization, and compensation in successful aging. In J. Brändstadter & R. M. Lerner (Eds.), *Action and development: Origins and functions of intentional self-development* (pp. 401–434). Thousand Oaks, CA: Sage.

Fried, L. P., Borhani, N. O., Enright, P., Furberg, C. D., Gardin, J. M., Kronmal, R. A., et al. (1991). The cardiovascular health study: Design and rationale. *Annals of Epidemiology, 1,* 263–276.

Friedman, L. J. (1999). *Identity's architect: A Biography of Erik H. Erikson,* New York: Simon & Schuster.

Fries, J. F. (1980). Aging, natural death, and the compression of morbidity. *New England Journal of Medicine, 303,* 130–135.

Fries, J. F. (1983). The compression of morbidity: Miscellaneous comments about a theme. *Gerontologist, 24,* 354–359.

Fries, J. F., & Crapo, L. M. (1981). *Vitality and Aging.* San Francisco: W. H. Freeman.

Furstenberg, A.-L. (2002). Trajectories of aging: Imagined pathways in later life. *International Journal of Aging and Human Development, 55*(1), 1–24.

Gallagher-Thompson, D., Dal Canto, P. G., Jacob, T., & Thompson, L. W. (2001). A comparison of marital interaction patterns between couples in which the husband does or does not have Alzheimer's disease. *Journals of Gerontology: Psychological and Biological Sciences, 56,* 140–150.

Gallagher-Thompson, D., & Steffen, A. M. (1994). Comparative effects of cognitive-behavioral and brief psychodynamic pyschotherapies for depressed family caregivers. *Journal of Consulting and Clinical Psychology, 62*(3), 543–549.

Gallagher, D., Breckenridge, J., Thompson, L., & Peterson, J. (1983). Effect of bereavement on indicators of mental health in elderly widows and widowers. *Gerontology, 38,* 565–571.

Gallo, L. C., Bogart, L. M., Vranceanu, A.-M., & Matthews, K. A. (2005). Socioeconomic status, resources, psychological experiences, and emotional responses: A test of the reserve capacity model. *Journal of Personality & Social Psychology, 88*(2), 386–399.

Gallup, G., Gallup, A., Shriver, J., McMurray, C., & Swirsky, M. (Eds.) (1985). *Religion in America, 50 years: 1935–1985.* Gallup Report No. 236. Princeton, NJ.

Gallup, G. H. (1997). *Spiritual beliefs and the dying process: A report on a national survey.* Princeton, NJ.

Gallup, G. Jr., & Jones, T. (2000). *The next American spirituality: Finding God in the twenty-first century.* Colorado Springs, CO: Cook Communications.

Gallup, G., Jr., & Lindsay, D. M. (1999). *Surveying the religious landscape: Trends in U.S. beliefs.* Harrisburg, PA: Morehouse Group.

Garner (2002). Psychodynamic work with older adults. *Advances in Psychiatric Treatment, 8,* 128–135.

Gartner, J. (1988). The capacity to forgive: An object relations perspective. *Journal of Religion and Health, 27,* 313–320.

Gatz, M., Fiske, A., Fox, L., Kaskie, B., Kasl-Godley, J. E. & McCallum, T. J., Wetherell, J. L. (1998). Empirically validated psychological treatments for older adults. *Journal of Mental Health and Aging, 4,* 9–46.

George, L. K. (2002). Research design in end-of-life research: State of science. *Gerontologist, 42,* 86–98.

George, L. K., & Gwyther, L. P. (1986). Caregiver well-being: A multidimensional examination of family caregivers of demented adults. *Gerontologist, 26,* 253–259.

Giambra, L. M., Arenberg, D., Zonderman, A. B., Kawas, C., & Costa, P. T. (1995). Adult life span changes in immediate visual memory and verbal intelligence. *Psychology & Aging, 10,* 123–139.

Goldberg, D., Bridges, K., Duncan-Jones, P., & Grayson, D. (1988). Detecting anxiety and depression in general medical settings. *British Medical Journal, 297,* 897–899.

Gomez, A. (2002). Gender and the HIV/AIDS pandemic. *Women's Health Journal, 2,* 3–7.

Goodwin, R. D. (2002). Anxiety disorders and the onset of depression among adults in the community. *Psychological Medicine, 32*(6), 1121–1124.

Gordon, S. M. & Thompson, S. (1995). The changing epidemiology of human immunodeficiency virus infection in older persons. *Journal of the American Geriatrics Association, 43,* 7–9.

Gorenstein, E. E., Papp, L. A., & Kleber, M. S. (1996). Cognitive behvaioral treatment of anxiety in later life. *Cognitive and Behavioral Practice, 6,* 305–320.

Greenfield, E. A., & Marks, N. F. (2004). Formal volunteering as a protective factor for older adults' psychological well-being. *Journal of Gerontology: Psychological and Social Sciences, 59*(5), S258–S264.

Guralnik, J. M., Fried, L. P., & Salive, M. E. (1996). Disability as a public health outcome in the aging population. *Annual Review of Public Health, 17,* 25–46.

Gutierrez, L. (1990). Working with women of color: An empowerment perspective. *Social Work, 35,* 149–154.

Gutierrez, L. (2004). Empowering African American women as informal caregivers: A literature synthesis and practice strategies. *Social Work, 49*(1), 97–108.

Gutmann, D. (1987). *Reclaimed powers: Toward a new psychology of men and women in later life.* New York: Basic Books.

Haight, B. K. (1988). The therapeutic role of structured life review process in homebound elderly subjects. *Journal of Gerontology, 43,* 40–44.

Haley, W. E., Larson, D. G., Kasl-Godley, J., & Neimeyer, R. A. (2003). Roles of psychologists in end-of-life care: Emerging models of pratice. *Professional Psychology: Research and Practice, 34*(6), 626–633.

Harlow, S. D., Goldberg, E., & Comstock, G. W. (1991). A longitudinal study of the prevalence of depressive symptomatology in elderly widowed and married women. *Archives of General Psychiatry, 48,* 1065–1068.

Harman, D. (1998). Extending functional life span. *Experimental Gerontology, 33,* 95–112.

Havighurst, R. J. (1961). Successful aging. *Gerontologist, 1,* 8–13.

Hepple, J. (2004). Psychotherapies with older people: An overview. *Advances in Psychiatric Treatment, 10,* 371–377.

Hebl, J. H., & Enright, R. D. (1993). Forgiveness as a psychotherapeutic goal with elderly females. *Psychotherapy, 39,* 658–667.

Herr, J. J., & Weakland, J. H. (1979). *Counseling elders and their families: Practical techniques for applied gerontology* (Vol. 2). New York: Springer.

Higbee, K. L. (1988). *Your memory: How it works and how to improve it* (2nd ed.). Saddle River, NJ: Prentice-Hall.

Hill, R. D., & Bäckman, L. (1995). The relationship between the mini-mental state examination and cognitive functioning in normal elderly adults: A componential analysis. *Age and Ageing, 24,* 440–446.

Hill, R. D., Bäckman, L., & Stigsdotter-Neeley, N. (2000). *Cognitive rehabilitation in old age.* New York: Oxford University Press.

Hill, R. D., Campbell, B. W., Foxley, D., & Lindsay, S. (1997). Effectiveness of the number-consonant mnemonic for retention of numeric material in community-dwelling older adults. *Experimental Aging Research, 14,* 207–211.

Hill, R. D., Evancovich, K. D., Sheikh, J., & Yesavage, J. A. (1987). Imagery mnemonic training in a patient with primary degenerative dementia. *Psychology & Aging, 2,* 204–205.

Hill, R. D., Grut, M., Wahlin, A., Herlitz, A., Winblad, B., & Backman, L. (1995). Predicting memory performance in optimally healthy very old adults. *Journal of Mental Health and Aging, 1*(1), 55–65.

Hill, R. D., Nilsson, L.-G., Nyberg, L., & Bäckman, L. (2003). Cigarette smoking and cognitive performance in healthy Swedish adults. *Age and Ageing, 32*(5), 548–550.

Hill, R. D., Packard, T., & Lund, D. (1996). Bereavement. In J. A. Sheikh (Ed.), *Treating the elderly* (pp. 45–74). San Francisco: CA: Jossey-Bass.

Hill, R. D., Thorn, B. L., Bowling, J., & Morrison, A. (2002). *Geriatric Residential Care.* Mahwah, NJ: Lawrence Erlbaum.

Hill, R. D., Thorn, B. L., & Packard, T. (2000). Counseling older adults: Theoretical and empirical issues in prevention and intervention. In S. D. Brown & R. W. Lent (Eds.), *Handbook of Counseling Psychology* (pp. 499–531). New York: John Wiley.

Hill, R. D., Wahlin, A., Winblad, B., & Bäckman, L. (1995). The role of demographic and life style variables in utilizing cognitive support for episodic remembering among very old adults. *Journal of Gerontology: Psychological Sciences, 50,* 219–227.

Hogan, D. B., Ebly, E. M., & Fung, T. S. (1999). Disease, disability, and age in cognitively intact seniors: Results from the Canadian Study of Health and Aging. *Journals of Gerontology: Biological and Medical Sciences, 54*(2), 77–82.

Holliday, S. G., & Chandler, M. J. (1986). Wisdom: Explorations in adult competence. In J. A. Meacham (Ed.), *Contributions to human development* (Vol. 17, pp. 1–96). Basel, Switzerland: Karger.

Holmes, T., & Rahe, R. (1967). The social readjustment scale. *Journal of Psychosomatic Research, 11*, 213–218.

Hopko, D., Stanley, M. A., Reas, D. L., Wetherell, J. L., Beck, G. L., Novy, D. M. et al. (2003). Assessing worry in older adults: Confirmatory factor analysis of the Penn State Worry Questionnaire and psychometric properties of an abbreviated model. *Psychological Assessment, 15*(2), 173–183.

Hubert, H. B., Bloch, D. A., Oehlert, J. W., & Fries, J. F. (2002). Lifestyle habits and compression of morbidity. *Journals of Gerontology: Biological and Medical Sciences, 57*(6), 347–351.

Hultsch, D. F., Hertzog, C., Small, B. J., & Dixon, R. A. (1999). Use it or lose it: Engaged lifestyle as a buffer of cognitive decline in aging? *Psychology & Aging, 14*(2), 245–263.

Hybels, C. F., Blazer, D. G., & Pieper, C. F. (2001). Toward a threshold for subthreshold depression: An analysis of correlates of depression by severity of symptoms using data from an elderly community sample. *Gerontologist, 41*(3), 357–365.

Hyer, L., Kramer, D., & Sohnle, S. (2004). CBT with older people: Alterations and the value of the therapuetic alliance. *Psychotherapy: Theory, Research, Practice, Training, 41*(3), 276–291.

Jacobs, S. C., Kasl, S. V., & Ostfeld, A. M. (1986). The measurement of grief. *The Hospice Journal, 2*, 21–36.

Jones, R. (2000). *Drug Treatment in dementia.* Malden, MA: Blackwell Science.

Jung, C. G. (1933). *Modern man in search of a soul.* Orlando, FL: Harvest.

Kane, R. A., & Kane, R. L. (1981). *Assessing the elderly: A practical guide to measurement.* Lexington, MA: Lexington Books.

Katz, S., Downs, T. V., & Grotz, R. C. (1970). Progress in the development of an index of ADL. *Gerontologist, 10*, 20–30.

Kausler, D. H. (1994). *Learning and memory in normal aging.* San Diego: Academic Press.

Kayser-Jones, J. (2002). The experience of dying: An ethnographic nursing home study. *Gerontologist, 42*, 11–19.

Kempen, G. I. J. M., Miedema, I., Ormel, J., & Molenaar, W. (1996). The assessment of disability with the Groningen Activity Restriction Scale: Conceptual framework and psychometric properties. *Social Science Medicine, 43*(11), 1602–1996.

Kemper, T. L. (1994). Neuroanatomical and neuropathological changes during aging and dementia. In A. L. Martin & J. E. Knoefel (Eds.), *Geriatric Neurology* (2nd ed., pp. 3–67). New York: Oxford University Press.

Kierkegaard, S. (1970). *The concept of dread.* Princeton, NJ: Princeton University Press.

Kinsella, K., & Velkoff, B. (2001). *An aging world: 2001*. Washington, DC: U.S. Census Bureau.

Kliegl, R. K., Smith, J., & Baltes, P. B. (1989). Testing-the-limits and the study of adult age differences in cognitive plasticity of a mnemonic skill. *Developmental Psychology, 25*, 247–256.

Kliegl, R. K., Smith, J., & Baltes, P. B. (1990). On the locus and process of magnification of age differences during mnemonic training. *Developmental Psychology, 26*, 894–904.

Knight, B. G. (1996). Psychodynamic therapy with older adults: Lessons from scientific gerontology. In R. T. Woods (Ed.), *Handbook of clinical psychology & aging* (pp. 545–573). Chichester, U.K., John Wiley & Sons.

Knight, B. G. (1996). *Psychotherapy with older adults*. Thousand Oaks, CA: Sage.

Koplan, J. P., & Fleming, D. W. (2000). Current and future public health challenges. *Journal of the American Medical Association, 284*, 1696–1699.

Kowaz, A. M., & Marcia, J. E. (1991). Development and validation of a measure of Eriksonian industry. *Journal of Personality & Social Psychology, 60*(3), 390–397.

Krach, C. A. & Velkoff, V. A. (1999). Centenarians in the United States: *Current population reports*. Bureau of the census U.S. Govt. Printing Office, Washington, DC (Document #: P23-199RV).

Kral, V. A. (1958). Neuropsychiatric observations in an old peoples home. Studies of memory dysfunction in senescence. *Journal of Gerontology, 13*, 169–176.

Kramer, D. A. (1990). Conceptualizing wisdom: The primacy of affect-cognition relations. In R. Sternberg (Ed.), *Wisdom: Its nature, origins and development* (pp. 279–309). Cambridge, U.K.: Cambridge University Press.

Krause, N., & Ellison, C. G. (2003). Forgiveness by God, forgiveness of others, and psychological well-being in late life. *Journal of the Scientific Study of Religion, 42*, 377–391.

Kübler-Ross, E. (1969). *On death and dying*. New York: Macmillan.

Kuehne, V. S., & Sears, H. A. (1993). Beyond the call of duty: Older volunteers committed to children and families. *Journal of Applied Gerontology, 12*, 425–438.

Kurland, N. D. (1982). The Scandinavian study circle: An idea for the US. *Lifelong Learning: The Adult Years, 30*, 25–27.

Kutza, E. A., & Keigher, S. M. (1991). The elderly "new homeless": An emerging population at risk. *Social Work, 36*(4), 288–293.

Landman, J. (1987). Regret: A theoretical and conceptual analysis. *Journal for the Theory of Social Behaviour, 17*, 135–160.

Lang, F. R., & Carstensen, L. L. (1994). Close emotional relationships in late life: Further support for proactive aging in the social domain. *Psychology & Aging, 9*, 315–324.

Langle, A. (2004). Objectives of existential psychology and existential psychotherapy: Answering Paul Wong's editorial. *International Journal of Existential Psychology and Psychotherapy, 1,* 99–102.

Langs, R. (2004). Death anxiety and the emotion-processing mind. *Psychoanalytic Psychology, 21*(1), 31–53.

Lantz, J. (1975). *Marital relationship perceptions test.* Columbus, OH: Lantz Counseling Associates.

Lantz, J., & Raiz, L. (2004). Existential psychotherapy with older adult couples: A five-year treatment report. *Clinical Gerontologist, 27*(3), 39–54.

Lawton, M. P., & Brody, E. M. (1969). Assessment of older people: Self-maintaining and instrumental activities of daily living. *Gerontologist, 9*(3), 179–186.

Lecci, L., Okun, M. A., & Karoly, P. (1994). Life regrets and current goals as predictors of psychological adjustment. *Journal of Personality and Social Psychology, 66,* 731–741.

LeDuff, C. (2003, July 17). Ten die after driver plows through outdoor California market. *The New York Times,* p. A1.

Lehman, D. R., Ellard, J. H., & Wortman, C. B. (1986). Social support for the bereaved: Recipients' and providers' perspectives on what is helpful. *Journal of Consulting and Clinical Psychology, 54,* 438–446.

LeShan, L. (1969). Psychotherapy and the dying patient. In L. Pearson (Ed.), *Death and dying: Current issues in the treatment of the dying person.* Cleveland, OH: Case Western Reserve University.

Leveille, S. G., Fried, L. P., McMullen, W., & Guralnik, J. M. (2004). Advancing the taxonomy of disability in older adults. *Journals of Gerontology: Biological and Medical Sciences, 59*(1), M86–93.

Levine, S. (1997, November 21). Creating an Eden for seniors: Nursing home movement stresses quality of life. *The Washington Post,* pp. 35–36.

Lichtenberg, P. A. (Ed.). (1999). *Handbook of assessment in clinical gerontology.* New York: Wiley.

Lichter, I., Mooney, J., & Boyd, M. (1993). Biography as therapy. *Palliative Medicine, 7*(2), 133–137.

Luborsky, B. R. (1994). The cultural adversity of physical disability: Erosion of full adult personhood. *Journal of Aging Studies, 8,* 239–254.

Luszcz, M. A., & Bryan, J. (1999). Toward understanding age-related memory loss in late adulthood. *Gerontology, 45,* 2–9.

Mackenzie, A., & Allen, R. P. (2003). Alcoholics' evaluations of alcoholism treatment. *Alcoholism Treatment Quarterly, 21*(2), 1–18.

Mahalik, J. R., Cournoyer, R. J., DeFranc, W., Cherry, M., & Napolitano, J. M. (1998). Men's gender role conflict and use of psychological defenses. *Journal of Counseling Psychology, 45,* 247–255.

Manton, K. G., Corder, L. S., & Stallard, E. (1997). Chronic disability trends in elderly United States populations: 1982–1994. *Proceedings of the National Academy of Sciences, 94,* 2593–2598.

Manton, K. G., & Saldo, B. J. (1992). Disability and mortality among the oldest old: Implications for current and future health and long term care service needs. In R. M. Suzman, D. P. Willis, & K. G. Manton (Eds.), *The oldest old* (pp. 199–250). New York: Oxford University Press.

Manton, K. G., & Waidmann, T. A. (1998). *International evidence on disability trends among the elderly.* (No. DHHS-100-97-0010). Washington, DC: U.S. Department of Health and Human Services.

Marsiske, M., Lange, F. R., Baltes, P. B., & Baltes, M. M. (1995). Selective optimization with compensation: Life-span perspectives on successful human development. In R. Dixon & L. Bäckman (Eds.), *Compensation for psychological deficits and declines: Managing losses and promoting gains* (pp. 35–79). Mahwah, NJ: Erlbaum.

Matt, G. E., Dean, A., Wang, B., & Wood, P. (1992). Identifying clinical syndromes in a community sample of elderly persons. *Psychological Assessment, 4*(2), 174–184.

Mattimore, T. J., Wenger, N. S., Cesbiens, N. A., Teno, J. M., Hamel, M. B., Liu, H. et al. (1997). Surrogate and physician understanding of patients' preference for living permanently in a nursing home. *Journal of the American Geriatrics Society, 45,* 818–824.

Mattis, S. (1988). *Dementia Rating Scale: Professional manual.* Odessa, FL: Psychological Assessment Resources.

Mattis, S. (1989). *Dementia Rating Scale.* Odessa, Florida: Psychological Assessment Resources.

May, R. (1967). *Psychology and the human dilemma.* New York: W. W. Norton.

May, R. (1983). *The discovery of being.* New York: Basic Books.

McCrae, R. R., Costa, P. T., Ostendorf, F., Angleitner, A., Hrebickova, M., Avia, M. D. et al. (2000). Nature of nurture: Temperment, personality, and life span development. *Journal of Personality & Social Psychology, 78*(1), 173–186.

McCullough, M. E., Emmons, R. A., & Tsang, J. (2002). The grateful disposition: A conceptual and empirical topography. *Journal of Personality & Social Psychology, 82*(1), 112–127.

Meichenbaum, D. (1996). Stress inoculation training for coping with stressors. *The Clinical Psychologist, 49,* 4–7.

Miller, W. R., & Thoresen, C. E. (2003). Spirituality, religion, and health: An emerging research field. *American Psychologist, 58*(1), 4–35.

Mitnitski, A. B., Graham, J. E., Mogliner, A. J., & Rockwood, K. (1999). The rate of decline in function in Alzheimer's disease and other dementias. *Journal of Gerontology, Biological and Medical Sciences, 54,* 65–69.

Mitrani, V. B., & Czaja, S. J. (2000). Family-based therapy for dementia caregivers: Clinical observations. *Aging and Mental Health, 4,* 200–209.

Mitrushina, M., & Satz, P. (1991). Reliability and validity of the mini-mental state exam in neurologically intact elderly. *Journal of Clinical Psychology, 47,* 537–543.

Mittelman, M. S., Epstein, C., & Pierzchala, A. (2002). *Counseling the Alzheimer's caregiver: A resource for health care professionals.* Chicago: American Medical Association.

Molinari, V. (1999). Using reminiscense and life review as natural therapeutic strategies in group therapy. In M. Duffy (Ed.), *Handbook of counseling and psychotherapy with older adults* (pp. 154–165). New York: John Wiley.

Molinari, V., & Reichlin, B. (1985). Life review reminiscence in the elderly: A review of the literature. *International Journal of Aging and Human Development, 20,* 81–92.

Morgan, A. C., & Goldstein, M. (2003). Psychodynamic psychotherapy with older adults. *Psychiatric Services, 54*(12), 1592–1594.

Morrow-Howell, N., Hinterlong, J., Rozario, P. A., & Tang, F. (2003). Effects of volunteering on the well-being of older adults. *Journals of Gerontology: Psychological and Social Sciences, 58*(3), 137–145.

Mundt, J. C., Freed, D. M., & Greist, J. H. (2000). Lay person-based screening for early detection of Alzheimer's disease: Development and validation of an instrument. *Journal of Gerontology: Psychological Sciences, 55*(3), 163–170.

Murrell, S. A., Meeks, S., & Walker, J. (1991). Protective functions of health and self-esteem against derpession in older adults facing illness or bereavement. *Psychology & Aging, 6*(3), 352–360.

Murrell, S. A., Norris, F., & Hutchings, G. (1984). Distribution and desirability of life events in older adults: Population and policy implications. *Journal of Community Psychology, 12,* 301–311.

Musick, M. A., Herzog, A. R., & House, J. S. (1999). Volunteering and mortality among older adults: Findings from a national sample. *Journals of Gerontology: Social Sciences, 54,* 173–180.

National Alzheimer's Association (1995). *Giving up the car keys.* National Newsletter, 15(3), 3–4.

National Center for Health Statistics (2004). *Health: United States.* Washington, DC: U.S. Government Printing Office.

National Institutes of Mental Health (2001). *The numbers count: Mental disorders in America, 2001.* Bethesda, MD, U.S. Dept. of Health & Human Services, National Institutes of Health. (NIH publ# 01-4584).

National Hospice and Palliative Care Organization (NHPCO). (2000). *Family member satisfaction with hospice care: 1994–2000.* Alexandria, VA. (http://www.nhpco.org): Author.

National Hospice and Palliative Care Organization. Alexandria, VA. (http://www.nhcpo.org) (2001). *NHPCO facts and figures:* Author.

Neitzsche, F. (1958). *Thus Spake Zarathustra.* New York: Random House.

Newman, A. B., Arnold, A. M., Naydeck, B. L., Fried, L. P., Burke, G. L., Enright, P., et al. (2003). "Successful aging": Effect of subclinical cardiovascular disease. *Archives of Internal Medicine, 163,* 2315–2322.

Niemeyer, R. A. (1988). Death anxiety. In H. Wass, R. Berardo & R. A. Neimeyer (Eds.), *Dying: Facing the facts* (2nd ed., pp. 97–136). Washington, DC: Hemisphere.

Niemeyer, R. A. (1994). *Death anxiety handbook: Research, instrumentation, and application.* New York: Taylor & Francis.

Niemeyer, R. A. (2001). *Meaning, reconstruction and the experience of loss.* Washington, DC: American Psychological Association.

Niemeyer, R. A., Wittokowski, J., & Moser, R. P. (2004). Psychological research on death attitudes: An overview and evaluation. *Death Studies, 28,* 309–340.

Norris, F., & Murrell, S. A. (1990). Social support, life events, and stress as modifiers of adjustment to bereavement by older adults. *Psychology & Aging, 5*(3), 429–436.

North, J. (1987). Wrongdoing and forgiveness. *Philosophy 62,* 499–508.

Nourhashemi, F., Andrieu, S., Gillette-Guonnet, S., Vellas, B., Albarede, J. L., & Grandjean, H. (2001). Instrumental activities of daily living as a potential marker of frailty: A study of 7,364 community-dwelling elderly women (the EPIDOS Study). *The Journals of Gerontology: Biological and Medical Sciences, 56,* 448–453.

Nusselder, W. J., Mackenbach, M. A., & Mackenbach, J. P. (1996). Rectangularization of the survival curve in the Netherlands. *Gerontologist, 36,* 773–782.

Oliver, L. P. (1990). Study circles: New life for an old idea. *Adult Learning, 2*(3), 20–23.

Olshansky, S. J., Carnes, B. A., & Cassel, C. (1990). In search of Methuselah: Estimating the upper limits to human longevity. *Science, 250,* 634–640.

Oman, D., Thoresen, C. E., & McMahon, K. (1999). Volunteerism and mortality among the community-dwelling elderly. *Journal of Health Pscyhology, 4*(3), 301–316.

Ong, A. D., Bergeman, C. S., & Bisconti, T. L. (2004). The role of daily positive emotions during conjugal bereavement. *Journal of Gerontology: Psychological Sciences, 59,* 168–176.

Osterweis, M., Solomon, F., & Green, M. (1984). *Bereavement: Reactions, consequences, and care.* Washington, DC: National Academy Press.

Ostir, G. V., Carlson, J. E., Black, S. A., Rudkin, L., Goodwin, J. S., & Markides, K. S. (1999). Disability in older adults: Prevalence, causes, and consequences. *Behavioral Medicine, 24*(4), 147–156.

Pandya, S. M. (2005). *Racial & ethnic differences in older adults in long-term care service use*. AARP Public Policy Institute, Fact Sheet #119, pp. 1–2. Washington, D.C.

Palmore, E. B. (1995). Successful aging. In G. L. Maddox (Ed.), *Encylcopedia of aging: A comprehensive resource in gerontology and geriatrics* (2nd Ed, pp. 914–915). New York: Springer.

Park, D. C. (1992). Applied cognitive aging research. In F. I. M. Craik & T. A. Salthouse (Eds.), *The handbook of aging and cognition* (pp. 449–493). Hillsdale, NJ: Lawrence Erlbaum.

Parmelee, P., Lawton, M., & Katz, I. (1998). The structure of depression among elderly institution residents: Affective and somatic correlates of physical frailty. *Journals of Gerontology: Biological Sciences and Medical Sciences, 53*(2), 155–162.

Paunonen, S. V. (2003). Big five factors of personality and replicated predictions of behavior. *Journal of Personality & Social Psychology, 84,* 411–424.

Pavot, W., & Diener, E. (1993). Review of the Satisfaction With Life Scale. *Psychological Assessment, 5*(2), 164–172.

Pavot, W., Diener, E., & Fujita, F. (1990). Extraversion and happiness. *Personality and Individual Differences, 11*(12), 1299–1306.

Perls, T. T. (1995). The oldest old. *Scientific American, 272,* 70–75.

Petersen, R., Smith, G., Waring, S. C., Ivnik, R. J., Tangalos, E. G., & Kikmen, E. (1999). Mild cognitive impairment: Clinical characterization and outcome. *Archives of Neurology, 56,* 303–308.

Peterson, R. C. (2000). Mild cognitive impairment or questionable dementia. *Archives of Neurology, 57,* 643–644.

Peterson, R. C., Stevens, J., Gangull, M., Tangalos, E. G., Cummings, J., & DeKosky, S. T. (2001). Practice parameter: Early detection of dementia: Mild cognitive impairment. *Neurology, 56,* 1133–1142.

Pfeiffer, E. (1975). A short portable mental status questionnaire for the assessment of organic brain deficit in elderly patients. *Journal of the American Geriatric Society, 23,* 433–441.

Poage, E. D., Ketzenberger, K. E., & Olson, J. (2004). Spirituality, contentment, and stress in recovering alcoholics. *Addictive Behaviors, 29,* 1857–1862.

Post, S. G., Underwood, L. G., Schloss, J. P., & Hurlbut, W. B. (2002). *Altruism and altruistic love: Science, philosophy, and religion in dialogue*. New York: Oxford University Press.

Powell, L. H., Shahabi, L., & Thoresen, C. E. (2003). Religion and spirituality: Linkages to physical health. *American Psychologist, 58*(1), 36–52.

Qualls, S. H. (2004). Psychotherapy with older adults. In D. R. Atkinson & G. Hackett (Eds.), *Counseling Diverse Populations* (3rd ed., pp. 240–254). Boston: McGraw-Hill.

Raimy, V. (1975). *Misunderstandings of the self.* San Francisco, CA: Jossey-Bass.

Rando, T. A. (1998). *How to go on living when someone you love dies.* New York: Lexington.

Rando, T. A. (2000). *Clinical dimensions of anticipatory mourning: Theory and practice in working with the dying, their loved ones, and their caregivers.* Champaign, IL: Research Press.

Ranney, M. (2003). El Portal Latino Alzheimer's Project: Model program for Latino caregivers of Alzheimer's disease-affected people. *Social Work, 48*(2), 259–271.

Rattenberg, C. S., & Stones, M. J. (1989). A controlled evaluation of reminiscence and current topics discussion groups in a nursing home context. *Gerontologist, 29,* 768–777.

Reed, D., Foley, D., White, L., Heimovitz, H., Burchfiel, C., & Masaki, K. (1998). Predictors of healthy aging in men with high life expectancies. *American Journal of Public Health, 88*(10), 1463–1468.

Regier, D. A., Boyd, J. H., Burke, J. D., Rae, D. S., Myers, J. K., & Kramer, M. (1988). One-month prevalence of mental disorders in the United States: Based on five epidemiologic catchment Area sites. *Archives of General Psychiatry, 45,* 1977–1986.

Reisberg, B., Ferris, S. H., de Leon, M. J., & Crook, T. (1982). The global deterioration scale (GDS): An instrument for the assessment of primary degenerative dementia (PDD). *American Journal of Psychiatry, 139,* 1136–1139.

Reisberg, B., Ferris, S. H., de Leon, M. J., & Crook, T. (1988). The global deterioration scale (GDS). *Psychopharmacology Bulletin, 24,* 661–663.

Remondet, J. H., & Hansson, R. O. (1987). Assessing a widow's grief—A short index. *Journal of Gerontological Nursing, 13*(4), 31–34.

Rentz, C., Krikorian, R., & Keys, M. (2004). Grief and mourning from the perspective of the person with a dementing ilness: Beginning the dialogue. *Omega, 50*(3), 165–179.

Rodeheffer, R. J., Gerstenblith, G., Becker, L. C., Fleg, J. L., Weisfeldt, M. L., & Lakatta, E. G. (1984). Exercise cardiac output is maintained with advancing age in healthy human subjects: Cardiac dilation and increased stroke volume compensate for a diminshed heart rate. *Circulation, 69*(2), 203–213.

Rogers, S. L., & Friedhoff, L. T. (1998). Long-term efficacy and safety of donepezil in the treatment of Alzheimer's disease: An interim analysis of the results of a U.S. multicentre open label extension study. *European Neuropsychopharmacology, 8,* 67–75.

Rosowsky, E. (1999). Couple therapy with long-married older adults. In M. Duffy (Ed.), *Handbook of counseling and psychotherapy with older adults* (pp. 242–266). New York: John Wiley.

Roth, A., & Fonagy, P. (2005). *What works and for whom? A critical review of psychotherapy research* (2nd ed.). New York: Guilford Press.

Rowe, J. W., & Kahn, R. L. (1987). Human aging: Usual and successful. *Science, 237,* 143–149.

Rowe, J. W., & Kahn, R. L. (1998). *Successful Aging.* New York: Pantheon Books.

Rozanski, A. & Kubzansky, L. D. (2005). Psychologic functioning and physical health: A paradigm of flexibility. *Psychosomatic Medicine, 67,* S47–S53.

Ruscio, A. M., Borkovec, T. D., & Ruscio, J. (2003). A taxometric investigation of the latent structure of worry. *Journal of Abnormal Psychology, 110*(3), 413–422.

Rye, M. S., Pargament, K. I., Ali, M. A., Beck, G. L., Dorff, E. N., Hallisey, V. N. et al. (2000). Religious perspectives on forgiveness. In M. E. McCullough, K. I. Pargament & C. E. Thoresen (Eds.), *Forgiveness: Theory, research, and practice* (pp. 17–40). New York: Guilford Press.

Ryff, C. D. (1982). Sucessful aging: A developmental approach. *Gerontologist, 22,* 209–214.

Sable, P. (1991). Attachment, loss of spouse, and grief in elderly adults. *Omega, 23,* 129–142.

Saddock, B. J., & Saddock, V. A. (2003). *Kaplan and Saddock's synopsis of psychiatry: Behavioral sciences clinical psychiatry.* Philadelphia, PA: Lippincott, Williams & Wilkins.

Salamon, M. J., & Conte, V. A. (1984). *Life Satisfaction in the Elderly Scale* (LSES). Odessa, FL: Psychological Assessment Resources.

Salive, M. E., & Guralnik, J. M. (1997). Disability outcomes of chronic disease and their implications for public health. In T. Hickey, M. A. Speers, & T. R. Prohaska (Eds.), *Public health and aging* (pp. 87–106). Baltimore, MD: Johns Hopkins University Press.

Salthouse, T. A. (1991). *Theoretical perspective in cognitive aging.* Mawah, NJ: Lawrence Erlbaum.

Salthouse, T. A. (2004). The what and when of cognitive aging. *Current Directions in Psychological Science, 13*(4), 140–144.

Sanchez-Ayendez, M. (1988). *Elderly Puerto Ricans in the United States.* New York: Greenwood Press.

Schaie, K. W. (1994). The course of adult intellectual development. *American Psychologist, 49,* 304–313.

Schaie, K. W. (1995). *Intellectual development in adulthood: The Seattle Longitudinal Study.* New York: Cambridge University Press.

Schaie, K. W. (2005). *Developmental influences on adult intelligence.* New York: Oxford University Press.

Schaie, K. W., Dutta, R., & Willis, S. L. (1991). Relationship between rigidity-flexibility and cognitive abilities in adulthood. *Psychology & Aging, 6,* 371–383.

Scheier, M. F., Carver, C. S., & Bridges, M. W. (2001). Optimism, pessimism, and psychological well-being. In E. C. Chang (Ed.), *Optimism and pessimism: Implications for theory, research, and practice* (pp. 189–216). Washington, DC: American Psychological Association.

Scholey, K. A., & Woods, B. T. (2003). A series of brief cognitive therapy interventions with people experiencing both dementia and depression: A description of techniques and common themes. *Clinical Psychology and Psychotherapy, 10*, 175–185.

Schultz, P. W., & Searleman, A. (2002). Rigidity of thought and behavior: 100 years of research. *Genetic, Social, and General Psychology Monographs, 128*, 165–207.

Schulz, R., Maddox, G. L., & Lawton, M. P. (Eds.). (2000). *Interventions research with older adults.* (Vol. 18). New York: Springer.

Schulz, R., O'Brien, A. T., Bookwala, J., & Fleissner, K. (1995). Psychiatric and physical morbidity effects of dementia caregiving: Prevalence, correlates, and causes. *Gerontologist, 35*, 691–771.

Schut, H. A., de Keijser, J., van den Bout, J., & Dijkhuis, J. H. A. R. (1991). Post-traumatic stress symptoms in the first years of conjugal bereavement. *Anxiety Research, 4*(1), 225–234.

Scogin, F., Rickard, H. C., Keith, S., Wilson, J., & McElreath, L. (1992). Progressive and imaginal relaxation training for elderly persons with subjective anxiety. *Psychology & Aging, 7*(3), 419–424.

Seeman, T. E., Charpentier, P. A., Berkman, L. F., Tinetti, M. E., Guralnik, J. M., Albert, M. et al. (1994). Predicting changes in physical performance in a high functioning elderly cohort: McArthur Studies of Successful Aging. *Journal Of Gerontology, 3*(49), 97–108.

Sehl, M. E., & Yages, E. F. (2001). Kinetics of human aging: rages of senescence between ages 30 and 70 years in healthy people. *The Journals of Gerontology: Biological and Medical Sciences, 56*, 198–208.

Seidlitz, L. (2001). Personality factors in mental disorders of later life. *American Journal of Geriatric Psychiatry, 9*, 8–21.

Seligman, M. E. P., & Csikszentmihalyi, M. (2000). Positive psychology: An introduction. *American Psychologist, 55*, 5–14.

Seta, J. J., McElroy, T., & Seta, C. E. (2001). To do or not to do: Desirability and consistency mediate judgements of regret. *Journal of Personality & Social Psychology, 80*(6), 861–870.

Shock, N. W., Greulich, R. C., Andres, R., Arenberg, D., Costa, P. T., Lakatta, E. G. et al. (1984). *Normal human aging: The Baltimore Longitudinal Study of Aging* (No. #84–2450). Washington, DC: National Institutes of Health.

Siegler, I. C., Poon, L. W., Madden, D. J., & Welsh, K. A. (1996). Psychological aspects of normal aging. In E. W. Busse & D. G. Blazer (Eds.), *The American psychiatric press textbook of geriatric psychiatry* (2nd ed., pp. 105–128). Washington, DC: American Psychiatric Press.

Small, S. A. (2001). Age-related memory decline: Current concepts and future directions. *Archives of Neurology, 58,* 360–364.

Springer, M. V., McIntosh, A. R., Winocur, G., & Grady, S. (2005). The relation between brain activity during memory tasks and years of education in young and older adults. *Neuropsychology and Aging, 19*(2), 181–192.

Stanley, M. A., Beck, J. G., Novy, D. M., Averill, P. M., Swann, A. C., Diefenbach, G. J. et al. (2003). Cognitive-behavioral treatment of late-life generalized anxiety disorder. *Journal of Consulting and Clinical Psychology, 71*(2), 309–319.

Stanley, M. D., & Novy, D. M. (2000). Cognitive-behavior therapy for generalized anxiety in late life: An evaluative overview. *Journal of Anxiety Disorders, 14*(2), 191–207.

Staudinger, U. M., Smith, J., & Baltes, P. B. (1992). Wisdom-related knowledge in a life review task: Age differences and the role of professional specialization. *Psychology & Aging, 7,* 271–281.

Steinhauser, K. E., Clipp, E. C., McNeilly, M., Chistakis, N. A., McIntyre, L. M., & Tulsky, J. A. (2000). In search of a good death: Observations of patients, families, and providers. *Annals of Internal Medicine, 132,* 825–832.

Stern, Y. (2002). What is cognitive reserve? Theory and research application of the reserve concept. *Journal of the International Neuropsychological Society, 8,* 448–460.

Sternberg, R. J. (1990). *Wisdom: Its nature, origins, and development.* Cambridge, UK: Cambridge University Press.

Steverink, N., Westerhof, G. J., Bode, C., & Dittmann-Kohli, F. (2001). The personal experience of aging, individual resources, and subjective well-being. *Journals of Gerontology: Psychological and Social Sciences, 56*(6), 364–373.

Stewart, M., Craig, D., MacPherson, K., Alexander, S. (2001). Promoting positive affect and diminishing loneliness of widowed seniors through a support intervention. *Public Health Nursing, 18,* 54–63.

Stroebe, M. S., Hansson, R. O., Stroebe, W., & Schut, H. (2001). *Handbook of bereavement research: Consequences, coping, and care.* Washington, DC: American Psychological Association.

Stroebe, W., & Stroebe, M. S. (1987). *Bereavement and health: The psychological and physical consequences of partner loss.* New York: Cambridge University Press.

Stroebe, W., & Stroebe, M. S. (1993). Determinants of adjustment to bereavement in younger widows and widowers. In M. S. Stroebe, W. Stroebe, & R. O. Hansson (Eds.), *Handbook of breavement* (pp. 208–226). New York: Cambridge University Press.

Stroebe, W., Stroebe, M., Abakoumkin, G., & Schut, H. (1996). The role of loneliness and social support in adjustment to loss: A test of attachment versus stress theory. *Journal of Personality & Social Psychology, 70,* 1241–1249.

Sulmasy, D. P. (2002). A biopsychosocial–spiritual model for the care of patients at the end of life. *Gerontologist, 42,* 24–33.

Tabbarah, M., Crimmins, E. M., & Seeman, T. E. (2002). The relationship between cognitive and physical performance: MacArthur studies of successful aging. *Journals of Gerontology: Biological and Medical Sciences, 57*(4), 228–235.

Tariot, P. N., Solomon, P. R., Morris, J. C., Kershaw, P., Lilienfeld, S., & Ding, C. (2000). A 5-month, randomized, placebo-controlled trial of galantamine in AD, *54,* 2269–2276.

Taylor, B. D., & Tripodes, S. (2001). The effects of driving cessation on the elderly with dementia and their caregivers. *Accident Analysis & Prevention, 33*(4), 519–528.

Templer, D. I. (1970). The construction and validity of a death anxiety scale. *Journal of General Psychiatry, 82,* 165–177.

Tennstedt, S., Cafferata, G. L., & Sullivan, L. (1992). Depression among caregivers of impaired elders. *Journal of Aging and Health, 4,* 58–76.

Thompson, L. W., Breckenridge, J. N., Gallagher, D., & Peterson, J. (1984). Effects of bereavement on self-perceptions of physical health in elderly widows and widowers. *Journal of Gerontology, 39,* 309–314.

Thorn, B. L. (2002). Defining residential care from a developmental perspective. In R. D. Hill, B. L. Thorn, J. A. Bowling, & A. Morrison (Eds.), *Geriatric Residential Care* (pp. 21–38). Mahwah, NJ: Lawrence Erlbaum.

Tombaugh, T. N. & McIntyre, N. J. (1992). The Mini-mental state examination: A comprehensive review. *Journal of the American Geriatric Society, 40,* 922–935.

Tomer, A., & Eliason, G. (1996). Toward a comprehensive model of death anxiety. *Death Studies, 20*(4), 346–365.

Trabert, M. L. (1996). Living in the moment: Support in the early stages of Alzheimer's disease. *Activities, Adaptation, and Aging, 20*(4), 1–20.

Turvey, C. L., Conwell, Y., Jones, M. P., Phillips, C., Simonsick, E., Pearson, J. L. et al. (2002). Risk factors for late-life suicide: A prospective community-based study. *American Journal of Geriatric Psychiatry, 10*(4), 398–406.

U.S. Census (2002). Special Populations Branch, Population Division. March, Washington, DC: U.S. Government Printing Office.

U.S. Census, (1997). *Statistical abstract of the United States: 117th edition.* Washington, DC: U.S. Government Printing Office.

U.S. Centers for Disease Control (2002). *HIV/AIDS surveillance report: U.S. HIV and AIDS cases reported through December 2001.* Atlanta, GA: Author.

U.S. Centers for Disease Control (2003). *Trends in aging—United States and worldwide.* Atlanta, GA: Author.

U.S. Dept. of Health and Human Services. (1999). *The Surgeon General's call to action to prevent suicide.* Washington, DC: Author.

U.S. Dept. of Health and Human Services. (2003). *Provider Education Article: Hospice care enhances dignity and peace as life nears its end.* (Program Memorandum). Washington, DC: Author.

Valliant, G. E. (2002). *Aging Well: Surprising guideposts to a happier life.* Boston: Little, Brown.

van Deurzen, E. (2002). *Existential counselling and psychotherapy in practice* (2nd ed.). London: Sage.

Van Willigen, M. (2000). Differential benefits of volunteering across the life course. *Journals of Gerontology: Psychological and Social Sciences, 55*(5), S308–318.

Verbrugge, L. M., & Jette, A. M. (1994). The disablement process. *Social Science Medicine, 38*(1), 1–14.

Verhaeghen, P., Geraerts, N., & Marcoen, A. (2000). Memory complaints, coping, and well-being in old age: A systemic approach. *Gerontologist, 40,* 540–548.

Watt, L., & Wong, P. A. (1991). A taxonomy of reminiscence and therapeutic implications. *Journal of Mental Health Counseling, 12,* 270–278.

Watt, L. M., & Cappeliez, P. (1995). Reminiscence interventions for the treatment of depression in older adults. In B. Haight & J. D. Webster (Eds.), *The art and science of reminiscing: Theory, research, methods and applications.* (pp. 221–232). Washington, DC: Taylor & Francis.

Webster, J. (1995). Adult age differences in reminiscence functions. In B. K. Haight & J. D. Webster (Eds.), *The art and science of reminiscing: Theory, research methods, and applications.* Bristol, PA: Taylor & Francis.

Weiss, R. S., & Richards, T. A. (1997). A scale for predicting quality of recovery following the death of a partner. *Journal of Personality & Social Psychology 72*(4), 885–891.

West, J. O. (1988). *Mexican-American folklore.* Little Rock, AR: August House.

West, R. (1985). *Memory fitness over 40.* Gainesville, FL: Triad.

West, R. L., Crook, T. H., & Barron, K. L. (1992). Everyday memory performance across the life span: Effects of age and noncognitive individual differences. *Psychology & Aging, 7,* 72–82.

Wetherell, J. L. (1998). Treatment of anxiety in older adults. *Psychotherapy: Theory, Research, Practice, Training, 35*(3), 444–458.

Wetherell, J. L., Gatz, M., & Craske, M. G. (2003). Treatment of generalized anxiety disorder in older adults. *Journal of Consulting and Clinical Psychology, 71*(1), 31–40.

Whitbourne, S. K., & Waterman, A. S. (1979). Psychosocial development during the adult years: Age and cohort comparisons. *Developmental Psychology, 15,* 372–378.

Whitbourne, S. K., Zuschlag, M. K., Elliot, L. B., & Waterman, A. S. (1992). Psychosocial development in adulthood: A 22-year sequential study. *Journal of Personality & Social Psychology, 63,* 260–271.

Williams, T. F., & Temkin-Greener, H. (1996). Older people, dependency, and trends in supportive care. In R. H. Binstock, L. E. Cluff & O. V. Merin (Eds.), *The future of long-term care* (pp. 51–71). Baltimore: MD: Johns Hopkins University Press.

Willis, S. L. (1985). Towards an educational psychology of the older adult learner: Intellectual and cognitive bases. In J. E. Birren & K. W. Schaie (Eds.), *Handbook of the psychology of aging* (pp. 818–847). New York: Van Nostrand-Reinhold.

Wilmoth, J. R. (1998). The future of human longevity: A demographer's perspective. *Science, 280*(5362), 395–397.

Wilson, R. S., Beckett, L. A., Bennett, D. A., Albert, M. S., & Evans, D. A. (1999). Change in cognitive function in older persons from a community population: Relation to age and Alzheimer's disease. *Archives of Neurology, 56,* 1274–1279.

Wisniewski, S. R., Belle, S. H., Coon, D. W., Marcus, S. M., Ory, M. G., Burgio, L. D. et al. (2003). The resources for enhancing Alzheimer's caregiver health (REACH): Project design and baseline characteristics. *Psychology & Aging, 18*(3), 375–384.

Wister, A. V. (2003). It's never too late: Healthy lifestyles and aging. *Canadian Journal on Aging, 22*(2), 149–150.

Witvliet, C. V. (2001). Forgiveness and health: Review and reflections on a matter of faith, feelings, and physiology. *Journal of Psychology and Theology, 29,* 212–224.

Wong, P. T. P. (2004). Existential psychology for the 21st century. *International Journal of Existential Psychology and Psychotherapy, 1,* 1–2.

Worden, J. W. (1991). *Grief counseling and grief therapy: A handbook for the mental health practitioner* (2nd ed.). New York: Springer.

Wortman, C. B., & Lehman, D. R. (1985). Reaction to victims of life crises: Support attempts that fail. In I. G. Sarason & B. R. Sarason (Eds.), *Social support: Theory, research, and applications* (pp. 463–489). Dordrecht, The Netherlands: Martinus Nijhoff.

Yalom, I. (1980). *Existential psychotherapy.* New York: Basic Books.

Yesavage, J. (1986). The use of self-rating depression scales in the elderly. In L. W. Poon (Ed.), *Clinical memory assessment* (pp. 214–217). Washington, DC: American Psychological Association.

Yesavage, J., Brink, T., Rose, T., Lum, O., Huang, O., Adey, V. et al. (1983). Development and validation of a geriatric depression screening scale: A preliminary report. *Journal of Psychiatric Research, 17,* 37–49.

Yong, H. H., Gibson, S. J., de L. Horne, D. J., & Helme, R. D. (2001). Development of a pain attitudes questionnaire to assess stoicism and cautiousness for possible age differences. *Journals of Gerontology: Psychological and Social Sciences, 56*(5), 279–284.

Zarit, S. H., Anthony, C. R., & Boutselis, M. (1987). Interventions with caregivers of dementia patients: Comparison of two approaches. *Psychology & Aging, 2*(3), 225–232.

Zarit, S. H. & Knight, B. G. (1996). *A guide to psychotherapy and aging: Effective clinical interventions in a life-stage context.* American Psychological Association, Washington: DC.

Zisook, S., & Shuchter, S. R. (1986). The first four years of widowhood. *Psychiatric Annals, 16,* 288–294.

INDEX

Index

Index

Index